PENGUI

Mid-Life Energy & Happiness

Gill Sanson is a Menopause Educator with the Family Planning Association in Auckland, New Zealand, and conducts regular workshops and seminars for mid-life women. She is a member of the Natural Food Commission and in recent years has been actively campaigning against the genetic modification of food. She has twice represented the Natural Law Party in parliamentary elections (both in the UK and New Zealand), has been a teacher of Transcendental Meditation for 25 years, and has had preliminary training in Ayur-Vedic medicine in India. Gill performs in a Javanese gamelan orchestra. She is married and has two adult children.

*For my sisters
Barbara and Julie
and my wonderful
women friends*

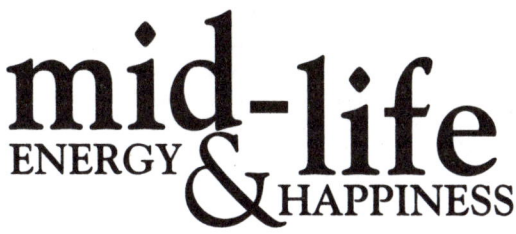

mid-life ENERGY & HAPPINESS

Live a Longer & Better Life

Gill Sanson

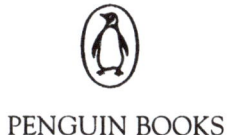

PENGUIN BOOKS

I am convinced that we can significantly improve our health and learn to live in harmony with our environment. I also believe everyone should be aware of the research and facts mentioned in this book which shed new light on the effects of environmental, nutritional and mind/body medicine. My intention is to inform and update so that you are in a better position to make choices. None of the suggestions or information is intended to be in any way prescriptive or replace the advice of a physician. Neither the publishers nor the author can accept responsibility for injuries or illness arising out of a failure by a reader to take medical advice.

PENGUIN BOOKS

Penguin Books (NZ) Ltd, cnr Airborne and Rosedale Roads, Albany,
Auckland 1310, New Zealand
Penguin Books Ltd, 27 Wrights Lane, London W8 5TZ, England
Penguin USA, 375 Hudson Street, New York, NY 10014, United States
Penguin Books Australia Ltd, 487 Maroondah Highway, Ringwood, Australia 3134
Penguin Books Canada Ltd, 10 Alcorn Avenue, Toronto, Ontario, Canada M4V 3B2
Penguin Books (South Africa) Pty Ltd, 4 Pallinghurst Road, Parktown,
Johannesburg 2193, South Africa

Penguin Books Ltd, Registered Offices: Harmondsworth, Middlesex, England

First published by Penguin Books (NZ) Ltd, 1999

1 3 5 7 9 10 8 6 4 2

Copyright © Gill Sanson, 1999

The right of Gill Sanson to be identified as the author of this work
in terms of section 96 of the Copyright Act 1994 is hereby asserted.

Designed by Mary Egan
Typeset by Egan-Reid Ltd
Printed in Australia by Australian Print Group, Maryborough

All rights reserved. Without limiting the rights under copyright reserved above,
no part of this publication may be reproduced, stored in or introduced
into a retrieval system, or transmitted, in any form or by any means
(electronic, mechanical, photocopying, recording or otherwise), without
the prior written permission of both the copyright owner and
the above publisher of this book.

CONTENTS

Acknowledgements		7
Foreword		9
Introduction		13
1	The Mid-life Challenge	21
2	Menopause	31
3	Ancient Wisdom in a Modern World	42
4	What Have They Done to Our Food?	58
5	Natural Plant Hormones	75
6	Natural Hormone Replacement	88
7	Osteoporosis	106
8	Breast Cancer	121
9	Women and Heart Disease	135
10	Depression at Mid-life	144
11	Minerals	158

| 12 | Secrets of a Long and Healthy Life | 169 |
| 13 | Natural Solutions for Common Symptoms of Menopause | 181 |

Recipes	192
References	209
Suggested Reading	221
Salute to the Sun	222
Index	225

ACKNOWLEDGEMENTS

Many people were helpful during the writing of this book. My thanks go firstly to the women who cheerfully offered their stories in order to reassure readers that they are not alone and that there are solutions to difficulties. In some cases names have been changed to protect identities.

Many thanks to Leslie Kenton for fuelling my passion for this subject, and generously writing the foreword for the book.

Many people have offered invaluable information and resources. In thanking them I must also make it clear that they were not asked to endorse the contents of this book in any way. The opinions expressed are mine alone. I am very grateful to Dr Helen Roberts, Research Manager, Family Planning Association (FPA), and Senior Lecturer in Women's Health at the School of Medicine, Auckland University; Dr Siriporn Chirawatkul, Medical Anthropologist, Khon Kaen University, Thailand; Dr Tessa Jones, Author and General Practitioner (Nutritional and Environmental Medicine); Mike Cushman, Pharmaceutical Compounding NZ Ltd; Dave Vousden, Efamol NZ Ltd; Jean Hughes and the Women's Health Action Trust; Dr Barbara Johnston, Jill Champness, and Amanda Sell.

Thanks to my friends: Gaynor Hamill for patiently editing the manuscript and for being so positive when I needed it most; Neil Hamill for help with legal issues; Linda Davy whose friendship and humour keeps me sane; Anne Thomson who provided information on favourable timing; Janet Hunt for her skilful input and moral support; my colleagues at FPA, in particular Cordelia Lockett, Vanesa Valentine, Diane Wilson and Jude Gillies; and Graeme and Raylene Lodge, Gail and Ken Pianta, Connie Clarkson, Kieran Garner, Janet Roxburgh and Jacqui Gallagher for their support and assistance.

My love and thanks to my wonderful family who have been so encouraging: my parents Joyce and Ken Gemmell, Barbara and Ross Johnston, Julie Gemmell and David Cooper, Geoff and Lorraine Gemmell, Aileen Sanson, and my son Jude, daughter Camille, and husband Stew for their input, patience and loving support.

FOREWORD

We are poised at the brink of a revolution in women's natural health care. This time, it is not pregnancy and natural childbirth that are its focus but attitudes and treatments given to women before, during and after menopause — including the use of drug-based oestrogens and progestins prescribed as HRT.

Once dazzled by high-tech medical intervention at birth, we willingly surrendered our bodies to epidurals, episiotomies and foetal monitoring equipment which promised pain-free trouble-free childbirth but too often delivered problems for mother and baby. Then, inspired by the work of visionary doctors such as Michele Odent, Pierre Vellay and Frederic Leboyer, more and more women began to insist on natural childbirth, breastfeeding and good mother–child bonding. We demanded the right to drug-free childbirth and control over our own bodies. Gradually — not without resistance — doctors, hospitals and government agencies have become more willing to provide it in response to the demands of ordinary women who believed or insisted there was a better way. It has been women themselves who brought to fruition the natural childbirth revolution just as now it is ordinary women who are issuing in the natural menopause revolution — a burgeoning movement to 'naturalise' women's reproductive and post-reproductive health.

Gill Sanson's practical and inspiring book *Mid-Life Energy and Happiness* is right at the forefront of women's demands for health and freedom as they come into full maturity spiritually, intellectually and emotionally. It is a book that is not only useful but visionary as well as superbly authoritative in its accuracy and research.

As Gill describes, a growing number of leading-edge health educators now vigorously challenge the wisdom of established medical practices in the treatment of women with drug-based hormones. They also object strongly to the widespread propaganda that accompanies the sale of HRT, claiming that the indiscriminate doling out of potent drug-based hormones can undermine a woman's fertility as well as trigger the development of menstrual agonies including PMS and menopausal miseries — from endometriosis to cancer of the breast and womb. This practice of making virtually every woman a 'patient' for most of her life by subjecting her to drug treatment not only where it may not be necessary but even when it can be potentially dangerous is a way of diminishing her personal power and taking away control over her own body.

Gill Sanson presents an alternative here. She sets out in clear and simple language the whole process of change that a woman goes through and explores all the important issues in depth with searing honesty: Is HRT appropriate? Are there other ways to deal with discomforts during the profound changes of menopause — from herbs to dietary change? How can the ancient practices of Ayur-Vedic medicine empower and make more graceful a woman's mid-life passage? What plants can help protect against osteoporosis, PMS, and menopausal difficulties? What do vitamins, minerals and other natural antioxidants have to offer in the prevention of premature ageing and the maximisation of energy? You will find it all within.

In other cultures, the transformation that takes place in a woman's life sometime between the ages of 35 and 60 has traditionally been considered a journey towards new freedom and power for a woman, a time of celebration where her creativity until

FOREWORD 11

then bound to her biology is at last set free for her to use as she wills. It is a time when women cease to give a damn what others think of their eccentricities and can set themselves free to soar into whatever realms they fancy. The passage we make at menopause — like the passage at birth or in giving birth — is a profound one which dissolves the boundaries of a woman's life and can take her deep inside on an archetypal heroine's journey to discover the real treasures of her life.

Each woman is biochemically and spiritually unique. So is the inner journey she must make if she is to succeed in her quest for wholeness. Such journeys need to be undertaken with the highest respect for the body, the spirit and the powers of nature which bring it about. Such journeys cannot be codified. They are not packaged holidays where you pay your money, take your anti-diarrhoea pills and know exactly what to expect. These, insist natural menopause revolutionaries, are journeys of the soul.

Gill Sanson has created some wonderful guidelines for any woman entering into the most profound passage she will ever go through.

Leslie Kenton

INTRODUCTION

It feels auspicious to have reached the middle of our lives at the end-point of the second millennium. We grew up and reached adulthood in the last 50 years of a century that has known change and technological advancement that was never dreamed of. Ours was the first generation not limited by the restrictions of wars and the legacy of the scars they leave. We bloomed and embraced the new world which emerged from the ashes of the Second World War. We are the baby boom generation — advantaged and liberated, we challenged the values of society and broke its boundaries.

We were the first generation to have access to the oral contraceptive pill. For the first time women could write their own biographies by choosing to delay or avoid child-rearing. This freedom added to the sense that we were somehow different, that we would change the world. We had rights and we would demand them. Our boundless personal expectations coincided with a surge of creative advancement world-wide which produced men on the moon, computer technology, advanced communication systems, micro-surgery, and finally biotechnology — the ability to modify and manipulate DNA.

The fallout from the catapult of humankind into the role of creator is only beginning to be apparent. Although brilliant individuals have gained mastery over some of the laws of nature, our inability to see or predict the full consequences of advancement means other vital laws are being violated and the planet is in crisis. Alarmingly, fertility levels are dropping world-wide, and the incidence of cancers has increased a staggering 50 per cent (in certain cancers by 300 per cent) in Western countries in the last 50 years.

Now the challenge is ours, and we have no choice but to respond to it. The human body is remarkably resilient and adaptable. But all the evidence suggests that our bodies are not managing to adapt rapidly enough to an environment that is now insidiously toxic. We have to understand the implications of the advancements of the last 50 years on our health and make crucial lifestyle and dietary adjustments not only to survive, but to lead a long and happy life. We need to evolve new strategies if we are to survive and continue to evolve as individuals and as a species.

There is good news. Knowledge revived from ancient classical systems of health care reveals effective disease-prevention strategies. Modern understanding of nutritional medicine and the subtle biochemical workings of the body bring more pieces of the puzzle together. We know better than ever before what is needed to survive and hopefully thrive despite environmental complications.

A GLOBAL PERSPECTIVE

Prior to this century only one out of ten people lived to the age of 65 years. In 1951 the world-wide life expectancy of a woman at birth was only 46 years. Women died early, often during childbirth or worn out from poor nutrition, repeated pregnancies and lactation. But due to improved nutrition, better living conditions and modern health care, by the year 2000 women can expect to live for 88 years.[1]

At birth a woman's life expectancy still exceeds that of men by seven years, even though women are still subject to more chronic diseases. In 1990 there were 467 million women in the world over the age of 50. It is predicted that by 2030 there will be 12,000 million and 23 per cent of these will be in China. The quality of life these women will experience is not known, because despite all the advantages of modern medicine and nutrition, a long life does not necessarily mean a healthy life.

While advancements in biochemistry and medical science have revealed knowledge that has resulted in this increased life expectancy, the understanding and application of these advances has also resulted in new diseases and unforeseen problems. A study published in the *Journal of the American Medical Association* in April 1998 documents that 106,000 people die each year in United States (US) hospitals from adverse drug reactions, and a further 2.2 million hospital patients have serious but non-fatal bad reactions to drugs. It can be estimated that the total cost of treating adverse drug events in the US is about $79 billion every year.[2, 3]

At the close of the century the realisation is dawning that much of what we thought was progress is in fact killing us. There have been huge mistakes for example thalidomide, Mad Cow Disease and diethylstilbestrol (DES). DES is a synthetic oestrogen given to an estimated 5 million pregnant women in the '50s and '60s to prevent miscarriages (it was later proven to have actually increased them). What resulted was a generation of daughters with higher than normal risk for cancers of the vagina and cervix, and sons with fertility problems and in some cases malformed genitals. Neither are we learning from the lessons of the past; the newest technological developments pose an even greater threat.

And despite the growth in understanding of human nutrition in the latter half of this century, there has been an unexpected and huge rise in the diseases of Western civilisation since the Second World War. Rampant diseases like coronary heart disease, diabetes and gallstones are being linked to the increase in fats and the reduction of health-promoting micro-nutrient and fibre-rich whole foods in the diet as a result of over-refining and processing.[4]

Cancer rates have escalated to epidemic proportions too. Since 1950 the overall cancer rates, adjusted for longevity of the population, have increased by nearly 50 per cent. Breast and colon cancers have increased by 60 per cent. Four decades ago the breast cancer rate was one woman in 20. Now it is one in nine. Breast cancer, the most common cause of death among women aged 40 to 50, is expected to continue increasing. Testes cancer in men has increased by 150 per cent and for men aged 28 to 35 by 300 per cent. Childhood cancers have increased by 20 per cent in the same period. Samuel Epstein, author of the prizewinning *Politics of Cancer* and co-author of *The Safe Shopper's Bible* and *The Breast Cancer Prevention Program*, claims that genetics has nothing to do with it. 'These are all results of avoidable exposures from carcinogens in consumer products, in the air, in water or in the workplace.'[5]

It is this peculiarly Western acceleration of disease that has led researchers to observe health patterns in Asian cultures. Asian women are generally much less at risk for breast cancer, heart disease and osteoporosis, and Asian men and women overall are much less at risk for the diseases that plague the Western world. Urban Asian women who have adopted more Western-style diets and consequently developed more of the risk factors for these diseases are now being urged to return to traditional Asian diets which are rich in calcium, digestive fibre, antioxidants and plant hormones or phytoestrogens. Asian women who immigrated to the US were found to lose the protection of these foods when they abandoned their traditional diet.[6]

Our soils are becoming depleted of essential minerals and trace elements after years of intensive chemical-assisted farming. Foods contain pesticide residues, are refined, processed, preserved with chemicals, and pre-cooked, losing much of their nutritional and antioxidant value. Finally and most frighteningly, foods are appearing on our supermarket shelves in a genetically modified form. Investigating what this means is horrifying. The DNA of plants is being altered to include the genes of animals, fish, bacteria, even viruses to produce plants that are capable of surviving a greater assault of pesticides and herbicides. These foods are not created in the interests of the consumer; they are for the benefit of the large corporations that produce them to make gargantuan profit. Most alarmingly, they have not been subjected to long-term testing for their effects on the public — the human guinea-pigs who now unknowingly ingest them.

The global environment is becoming increasingly permeated with industrial chemical contaminants. In 1940, one billion pounds of industrial chemical were created world-wide and in 1988 the figure was 600 billion pounds. The air we breathe, our waterways and soils are so polluted that we cannot avoid ingesting and absorbing chemicals from plastics, electrical components (PCBs), petrol, DDT residues, pesticides and herbicides, industrial cleaners, and household chemical products that are known to be hazardous to human health. New Zealand currently has a permissible level of hormone weed-killer in its drinking water that is 300 times as much as the European Union allows in its water.[7]

The illusion that New Zealand is clean and green is shattered. Our health statistics are frightening. We have the highest rate of childhood asthma in the Western world. One in six women have asthma. Our rates of osteoporosis, cardiovascular disease, and cancer are among the highest in the world. Breast cancer kills an estimated 600 women a year making it the major cause of death from cancer for women. Maori and Pacific Island women are four times more at risk for heart disease and lung cancer than non-Maori or Pacific Island women. They are also more at risk for asthma and cervical cancer.

Fertility levels are dropping world-wide too — clearly linked to hormone-mimicking herbicides and pesticides, PCBs (which permeate the planet so deeply now that they are being found in the fat cells of seals and whales in the Arctic), and DDT residues. The rapid rise in reproductive disorders world-wide is believed to be related to these pollutants. In a powerful statement in a recent address, the medical practitioner and researcher responsible for alerting women to the benefit of natural hormone replacement, Dr John Lee, said that the last generation of children who will be able to reproduce with ease may already have been born.

It is utterly crucial that we are all aware of the environmental issues and seek to take responsibility *en masse* for forcing change. As the mothers and the nourishing force in the world it is our challenge — we have to take action to ensure the survival of the earth and with it our children's children. It will be a contribution to humankind akin to that of our fathers and grandfathers in the world wars. They fought for their countries; we must now fight for the survival of the planet.

Individually we have to take responsibility for our health, our happiness and our spiritual welfare. Nature provides solutions. If we attune ourselves to living more in accord with the laws and rhythms of nature, we will achieve the health and wholeness we desire. Science also provides answers. The last decade has witnessed unprecedented growth in understanding the body's biological secrets. One of the most significant is the breakthrough in the understanding of free radicals and the damage these molecular 'terrorists' can do to our health. Free radicals are unstable oxygen molecules, which cause physical damage to cells during chemical reactions to replace their 'missing electron'. Every cell in the body sustains thousands of free radical 'hits' every day.

Free radicals have been identified as a major cause of many of the most serious chronic and degenerative diseases that accelerate ageing and ill health. Not only do our bodies generate free radicals, our environment is awash with them. We are exposed to ever-increasing quantities of free radicals as our lifestyles become further divorced from the conditions enjoyed by earlier civilisations. Free radicals are generated by eating fatty foods, which increases levels of dangerous oxidised lipids in our blood, leading to arteriosclerosis. Chemicals, preservatives and peroxides in food increase free-radical levels. So do ultra-violet radiation from the fierce Southern Hemisphere sunlight, microwaves, X-rays and magnetic fields. Even our houses aren't safe — residues from chemicals used in the manufacture of furniture, coverings or coatings on the walls and floor are all emitting free radicals as the chemicals break down with time. Cigarette smoking produces one of the most dangerous free-radical compounds we might ever take into our systems, and motor-vehicle emissions are another potent source. Stress and excessive exercise increases the free-radical assault on our bodies.

Exciting progress is being made daily as researchers identify the means to reverse this damage through the action of antioxidants. The answers are simple and all around us, and may have been known for millenia. Fruits and vegetables are a rich source of antioxidants, as are various vitamins such as A, C and E, and minerals such as zinc and selenium. But according to many studies, the most effective response to the free-radical challenge comes from the world's oldest system of natural health care, Ayur-Veda. The revival of ancient traditional plant formulas from India, which have been subjected to rigorous scientific scrutiny, has revealed antioxidants of unprecedented potency. These are discussed in subsequent chapters. We know better than ever before what we need to do, not only to live longer, but to enjoy energy, clarity and fulfilment with advancing years.

Mid-life for women is a transition that by its very nature demands that we change. It is a crucial rite of passage from which we emerge as wise, liberated women in our communities. Our reproductive function has ceased, and in most cases our children are grown; our intense child-rearing days are over. We are no longer at the mercy of fluctuating hormone levels. Provided we achieve a balance of healthy mind and body, mid-life marks a passage to a new adulthood where we can follow our own passions and interests, and achieve the personal potential we sensed in our childhood. The mid-life journey is one of self-discovery that leads to individual freedom, and in transforming ourselves, we transform the world around us. This book brings a blend of the wisdom of ancient civilisations and the advancements of modern scientific understanding, which together provide a recipe for the health and long life that is our birthright. What follows is a summary of essential traditional and modern health-care wisdom for quality of life far beyond the year 2000.

1
THE MID-LIFE CHALLENGE

Let us go forward into dancing and laughter, assuming a longer and better life.

Rig-Veda

Somewhere around the 48- to 50-year mark, many women find themselves experiencing a deep internal shift and it can stop them in their tracks. Without warning their previously predictable bodies take on off-beat primal rhythms, and emotions often follow suit. Their comfortable world appears to be disintegrating as a major life transition begins.

Change is normal — it is at the basis of all growth and evolution. It is the mechanism through which we move to new stages in life. New growth is often associated with loss of the familiar and it can bring with it fear of the unknown. By understanding the process and adapting to new ways of functioning, change becomes a mechanism for self-development.

Nature provides us with a new beginning when we pass through menopause and the mid-life transition. What can seem to be an alarming dismantling of the normal and the familiar is in fact an enormously significant passage to a new state of wisdom and wholeness. The change in our bodies forces change in our perception. We can no longer get away with abusing our bodies through wrong eating and lack of exercise, for example; neither can we indulge in an excessive lifestyle without immediate repercussions.

The mid-life transition is a gift which offers the opportunity for huge personal growth. It challenges us to ignore the pressures of a society that favours youth, and to value ourselves instead. It teaches us to confront our personal fears and renew our self-respect. It is a time to invest in our on-going good health through lifestyle adjustments, new researched therapies, and time-tested traditions. If we accept the challenge and adapt, we emerge liberated from outdated cultural restrictions and the limitations of hormonal fluctuations into an exciting and fulfilling new stage of life.

In her book *New Passages* Gail Sheehy writes: 'Menopause is a biological marker that demands women recognize where they are in life . . . It is an initiation into Second Adulthood. Women who take the time to evaluate where they are, physically, psychologically, spiritually, are the ones who will move ahead; they'll be more balanced and productive in their fifties and sixties.'[1]

It is also our generation's role to challenge outmoded attitudes to ageing, particularly the place of older women in society. Women aged 50 at the year 2000 can expect to enjoy at least 35 years of active life after mid-life and menopause. Rather than having fulfilled their biological purpose and outlived their usefulness, these women are a powerful resource of wisdom and energy which can be directed towards correcting the mistakes of the past and making the world a nourishing environment for future generations.

Studies and experience have shown that once through the menopause transition and into their fifties, women begin to take off. Many report that they have gained an inner harmony, and a greater sense of fulfilment and well-being than at any other stage of their lives. They feel fitter and healthier too because they now give more time and attention to taking care of themselves. Anthropologist Margaret Mead, surprised by how great she felt, coined the term 'post-menopausal zest'.

A TIME OF LIBERATION

Mid-life can be a journey of self-discovery, a realisation that valuing the self is primary, and that negative cultural attitudes are inconsequential. Women often report that they can freely express themselves at last and have acquired a liberating lack of concern for other people's opinion of them. Some experience the emergence of new skills they didn't know they had. Others desire to live an entirely new lifestyle. Many feel more in tune with their intuition and begin to pursue paths of self-development like meditation and yoga.

MID-LIFE CONFUSION

The major task is to successfully negotiate the transition through menopause — primarily by understanding it. Most of us lack education of this most significant life passage and are consequently daunted by it. It can coincide with other milestones and weighty responsibilities, which may direct our attention away from our own needs. We also become aware that we are moving into the risk category for major diseases and feel uncertain what to do to avoid them.

At this time of our lives we are usually still locked in the role of caregivers to our immediate families, often with the addition of elderly failing parents. We find it difficult to make our own needs a priority. Economic pressure and looming retirement require us in many cases to be working full-time. Children usually leave home at this time, which can be a big adjustment, and children leaving home and coming back again — a common phenomenon these days — is reported to be even more stressful!

Primary relationships sometimes falter now, or may have done already, and some women can find themselves alone for the first time in years. Throw menopause with its associated hormonal fluctuations into the equation and it can amount to a difficult life transition.

THE INVISIBLE WOMAN

Women often feel a deep desire for time out and solitude at mid-life, but find themselves caught on a treadmill of responsibilities in a world that doesn't understand. Many describe a psychological 'low' during their mid- to late forties. Although menopause brings freedom from the influence of the monthly cycle, and relief that unwanted pregnancy is no longer a possibility, for many it raises major issues about the physical and social consequences of growing older.

'I have always loved having birthdays and made the most of them. But this year, I turned 47 with a sense of dread, a very real feeling that the best years were over for me. I couldn't celebrate — I went and bought a new outfit to console myself and found it hard to look in the mirror.' Barbara is a beautiful, fit, highly intelligent woman. She has a great career, has successfully raised her children and has every reason to feel optimistic about her future.

Ours is a culture that worships youth and its associated beauty and fertility. It is common to feel quite suddenly 'invisible' in a world that festoons its billboards and magazines with the bodies and faces of the young.

'I am not noticed any more. I had to assert myself to keep my place in the queue at the bank this week when some young self-absorbed executives pushed past me,' said one woman. Others lament the passing of the days when they would turn heads on the street, and the ease with which they used to fall deliciously in and out of love.

THE PROMISE OF ETERNAL YOUTH

A huge industry has built up around keeping us looking young. We are exhorted to try creams, beauty treatments, and even 'corrective' surgery to stave off the dreaded and unthinkable ageing process. The underlying message is a damning one — older women are not valued.

The magazine stands at the supermarket checkout tell it all:

'She is 70. Her secret revealed.' (Picture of gorgeous older woman.)
'Best anti-ageing diet.'
'Diana's Race Against Time.'
'Do women have a use-by date?'
'The most age-defying beauty buys.'

As superficial as all this may seem, it is made additionally difficult because ours has not been a culture that actively values the rich intangibles that replace youth — wisdom and experience. Previous generations of women have not automatically risen to positions in society that reflect their life experience and provide good role-modelling and a source of wisdom for the young. Women have been increasingly unemployable after the age of 50.

CULTURAL ATTITUDES TO AGEING AND MENOPAUSE

In her book *Women's Bodies, Women's Wisdom*, Christiane Northrup writes: 'In our ageist culture, many women, instead of believing in their capacity to remain strong, attractive, and vital throughout their lives, instead come to expect their bodies and minds to deteriorate with age.'[2] The reverse is also the case. Not surprisingly, research shows that where the cultural expectation is to live a long life, individuals integrate that expectation and do live longer. Their bodies respond accordingly. They literally slow the ageing process to conform to cultural expectations.

Studies have shown that the psychological impact of menopause is influenced by how much a society values the older woman. Some cultures don't even have a word in their language for menopause. In societies like Papua New Guinea where women enjoy increased status as they age and where their communities have positive attitudes to ageing and the menopause, there are few if any uncomfortable symptoms. They look forward to this time of life.[3,4]

In Rajasthan in India, women who have been heavily veiled through their fertile years are able to take the veils off at menopause and are free to chat with the men in their villages. Understandably they view this new phase as immensely liberating and likewise have no difficulties at menopause. In the typical Indian household there are daughters or daughters-in-law who take over domestic responsibilities for the older woman who assumes lighter duties while she manages her way through menopause.

In a study conducted in Botswana, Africa, in 1990, in-depth interviews were conducted with twenty-five 50-year-old rural and urban women. The interviews revealed that the women viewed menopause positively. They saw it as a natural occurrence over which only God had control, a relief from menstrual bother and expenses, and freedom from unplanned pregnancy. Most interestingly and in direct contrast with the experience of the majority of Western women, most of the women experienced an increased libido or sex drive. Neither was menopause a tabu subject. The women readily sought help and information from older relatives and nurses.[5]

TIMES ARE CHANGING

Hearteningly, in a very recent survey of 1000 German women aged between 50 and 70 years it was found that the biggest concern over the physical changes of ageing was not physical attractiveness, weight gain or loss of figure, but rather loss of energy and vitality. Having good health rated far higher for these women than sex appeal. It was also noted that those with the most positive attitude to ageing had the least discomfort with their menopause.[6]

A New Zealand survey of 445 women ranging in age from 35 to 60 years was conducted in Christchurch in 1988. The women were surveyed for happiness at mid-life by measuring their overall health, their lifestyle and their attitude to life as they grew older. The majority of women, about 90 per cent, were very positive about their current life and their future. The percentage who were not so happy said it was mainly because of pain and discomfort due to menopause.[7]

EVERYONE AGES DIFFERENTLY

The ageing process is as individual as personality itself. What we present to the world is the sum total of the genetic, cultural, lifestyle, environmental, nutritional, physical and psychological influences of our lives. But it is our mental health that most influences how well we age. It is now known that people with good mental health transfer this to their bodies. Joyful, stimulated, relaxed individuals are more likely to be well and not be at risk for major illness. We are all subjected to stress in varying degrees at different times. But it is not the stress that makes us sick — it is our interpretation of it and our inability to adapt to it. Knowing this, it is possible to see why doing what you love to do and leading a healthy lifestyle can delay or even reverse the ageing process.

FACTORS THAT SLOW THE AGEING PROCESS

The following are factors known to slow the ageing process:
- Regular meditation or relaxation
- Nutrient- and antioxidant-rich diet
- Regular exercise
- Happy marriage or long-term relationship
- Job satisfaction
- Feeling of personal happiness
- Ability to laugh easily
- Ability to make and keep close friends
- Regular daily routine
- Taking regular holidays
- Feeling in control of personal life
- Enjoying leisure time, satisfying hobbies
- Ability to express feelings easily
- Optimism about the future
- Feeling financially secure, living within means[8, 9, 10, 11, 12]

CHRONOLOGICAL AND BIOLOGICAL AGE — WHAT IS THE DIFFERENCE?

There can be a big difference between chronological age and biological age. Chronological age is the number of years a person has lived. Biological age is an indication of a person's overall state of health compared to population averages. When testing biological age, standard measures of blood pressure, auditory (hearing) threshold, and near-point vision are used to compare it with chronological age.

As a hypothetical example, let's consider two 50-year-old women. Fleur is divorced, suffers from anxiety, smokes, feels lonely, eats poorly and takes little exercise. Marianne, on the other hand, is content with her personal relationships, feels healthy, exercises regularly, loves her job and her leisure activities. Because Fleur has negative influences dominating her life, her body when measured biologically is likely to be close to 10 years older and will be ageing quickly. Marianne, on the other hand, will be physically fit and could have the biological age of a woman at least five years younger.

A fundamental factor in the ageing process is wear and tear from stress and chronic fatigue. Nature's healing mechanism is rest. Many of us fail to achieve a healthy daily balance of rest and activity; neither do we deliberately structure effective relaxation strategies into our day. Providing the mind and body with regular deep rest automatically restores a normal natural state of balance.

The healing effect of profoundly deep rest has been verified by extensive research into the simple technique of Transcendental Meditation (TM). Studies have revealed that individuals who have been practising the technique for 20 minutes twice a day for five or more years use hospital services 50 per cent less and have an average biological age 12 years younger than their chronological age. A finding that particularly impressed the team of researchers was that older people showed results that were as good as younger people. That means a typical 60-year-old meditating five years or more would have the physiology of a 48-year-old.[13]

NUTRITIONAL MAGIC

Meeting our daily nutritional requirements is essential. Japanese women have the highest life expectancy in the world and their longevity is linked to their diet. It is now believed that the main reason for their low incidence of breast cancer, heart disease and hip fractures is their low-fat, high-fibre diet rich in minerals, vitamins, antioxidants and plant (phyto) hormones. They consume an abundance of fresh fruit and vegetables, legumes and whole grains and seafood. Ancient traditional herbs and treatments have an important role. Ginseng, for example, has been used for over 4000 years for longevity, infertility and impotence.

There is much literature and new thinking regarding the effects of free-radical damage on the ageing process. It is now believed that free radicals are responsible for over 100 diseases of the human body, and that if their activity can be neutralised or restrained, we will remain healthy and enjoy a full life for much longer. Although the body produces its own antioxidants, they are not sufficient to combat the onslaught of free radicals created by the 1990s' environment. Antioxidants are found in plants and enter our bodies via food. Not surprisingly, fruit and vegetables are the richest source.

How much we eat is important too. We now know that by eating less each day and only eating when we are hungry, we can slow the ageing process considerably. Animal studies have shown that restricting the diet of rodents leads to a 30 per cent increase in life span.[14] The islanders on Okinawa in Japan have more citizens over the age of 100 than any other population. They eat 17–40 per cent fewer calories than other Japanese, and have 30–40 per cent less heart disease, stroke, cancer, diabetes, and age-related disease.[15]

REVOLUTION

Thankfully, a change is taking place in our culture. A new revolution is afoot, and it is powered by the knowledge that we have control of our health and our destiny, and that the secrets for a long and healthy life are simple ones that have always existed in nature. Our vision of possibilities has shifted to include the wisdom of ancient traditions in conjunction with modern medicine, and the powerful effects of meditation, regular exercise, a nutritionally complete diet, and an avoidance of the hazards of the environment.

2
MENOPAUSE

Nothing in life is to be feared. It is only to be understood.
Marie Curie

Most of us who grew up in New Zealand learned little about menopause from our mothers or other women. It has been shrouded in silence, myth and misinformation, and the unspoken message has been to dread it. Yet it need not be feared. It is as natural as puberty, pregnancy and childbirth, and happens to all women. Fortunately attitudes are changing as the new generation of mid-life women confront and demystify it.

Somewhere between our early and our late forties, most of us begin to notice changes in our menstrual cycle. It usually becomes irregular and less predictable time-wise, but bleeding may become heavier or possibly lighter. In most cases it is manageable, but what takes many of us by surprise is that we feel physically and mentally so different.

'I woke up one morning and felt I had had a personality change. I felt tired and apathetic. Unbelievably, I lacked the confidence to make the smallest decisions — even down to what to have for dinner! I have always managed to do about ten things at once.' Jenny was lamenting her loss to a group in a menopause education session. Everyone was sympathetic. 'I have always run my own business and been able to make multiple decisions under stress,' added Pru. 'I was on my way home the other day and crashed the car. It wasn't serious, but I had to call a breakdown truck. Faced with a choice of who to call, I fell apart, felt paralysed. I had to get my daughter to deal with it. I was mortified!'

Menopause is different for everyone, and the possible experiences are widely varied. Some women (about 20 per cent) notice nothing at all, other than the end of their menstruating life. The rest of us are aware that big changes are afoot, and about 20 per cent have severe, even disabling symptoms of hormonal imbalance. The most common experience is the hot flush and its close relative night sweats, which can vary in intensity from woman to woman. Both are bothersome and even overwhelming at times. Rarely, women even report that hot flushes are so severe that their legs buckle under them. The sudden need to remove layers of clothes can occur at inappropriate times too — but necessity usually triumphs. Sadly, many women feel acutely embarrassed about their flushes and try to hide the fact that they have them.

We've been accustomed to the challenges of premenstrual syndrome (PMS), and although some menopause symptoms are similar, it presents new mental, physical and emotional developments. Some of the generally agreed signs of menopause are quite unusual and would seem to be unrelated to menopause unless you are aware of them. There are excellent and effective strategies to deal with difficulties, and knowing and understanding what is normal helps to reduce the impact.

Physical Signs
Hot flushes
Night sweats
Dry vagina
Headaches
Joint pain
Fatigue

Racing heartbeat
Creepy skin sensation
Clumsiness
Feeling of light-headedness
Dizziness
Disturbed sleep patterns

Psychological Signs
Mood swings
Tenseness
Anxiety
Depression
Irritability
Poor memory
Lower libido or sex drive
Difficulty concentrating and making decisions
Tearfulness
Loss of confidence
Difficulty coping
Panic attacks
Fuzzy thinking
Mental vagueness
(See Chapter 13 for treatment of these symptoms.)

It looks alarming when you see all the signs together, but be reassured that no one woman gets all of these symptoms — and certainly never at once! Some women have a mild occurrence of one or two only. And a lot of the experiences are interrelated. Night sweats can severely interrupt sleep patterns. Fatigue can reduce our coping abilities, and our concentration and decisiveness. Libido is an indicator of overall well-being too and is definitely influenced by lack of sleep as well as hormonal changes.

Memory loss can be a surprising symptom. Unless you know that it is due to the menopause transition and that it will therefore pass in time, it can be quite devastating and be wrongly interpreted as the beginning of the slippery slope into age-related amnesia. It can manifest as general forgetfulness (you find you have put the hairdryer in the fridge or you can't remember a friend's name when you go to introduce her) or it can be like mentally falling into a black hole where you cannot recollect what you were saying seconds before.

It is often hilarious in retrospect, but when you are working and need to be fully functional it can also be terrifying. Georgia found herself becoming quite inventive. 'I started to find myself calling people who were recognisable to me when they answered the phone but I had no idea why I had called them! So I would say things like, "Look I really need to talk to you but I have just had an international call come through, I'll call you back."'

Carol had always been able to rely utterly on her memory, and her family did as well, so when she woke up to find her car gone and declared it stolen, no one doubted her. The police were called, friends involved, and a major drama ensued until she remembered suddenly at the end of the day that she had left it at her workplace the day before. She was totally shocked by the experience and her confidence in her mental faculties shaken.

Edith's family thought she was going mad, and she was about ready to agree with them. She had changed completely — was forgetful, vague and often weepy. But the awful thing was that when she got into bed at night, something was creeping on her skin. She began to lie in wait for it in the dark and when it started she would switch on the light to catch it. There was never anything there, and the creepiness didn't respond to creams or washing. She attended a menopause education course and when the realisation dawned that she wasn't alone with her experience and that this was all a normal indicator of menopause her relief was enormous.

Understanding four things is vital:
1. Menopause is different for everyone.
2. There is a wide range of normal menopausal experience.
3. It is a transition that passes.

4. There are many simple and effective ways to ease the passage.

MENOPAUSE AND DEPRESSION

There is on-going debate about whether menopause and depression are linked, and it is generally agreed that they are not. It is known that there is no link between hormone levels and depression; neither is there any evidence that hormone replacement therapy (HRT) will help depression.[1]

In fact, women at mid-life are more likely to report positive moods than negative moods.[2] It is nevertheless true that women who have had a history of depression could re-experience it at this time. Many women report a 'bleakness' that descends from nowhere, lasts a day or two and lifts just as unpredictably. While clinical depression and menopause are no longer linked, previous generations of mid-life women in New Zealand were regularly treated with Valium (and became addicted to it). Many women were even hospitalised at mid-life, and my grandmother was one of these. Not fully understanding, I grew up with the expectation that I would most probably develop some form of mental instability at menopause.

But my wonderful piano-playing grandmother who recovered and returned to her family had other factors in her life that may have brought on her depression. She was permanently disabled by polio when a young mother, leaving her unable to walk without the aid of a walking stick. She brought up four children through the years of the Great Depression in the 1930s, which delivered enormous financial and emotional strain to people's lives.

Depression is most common in women in their thirties in New Zealand. It is now known that clinical disorders, including depression, continue to drop off in older women. However, at menopause those women who have a previous history of depression, who are less financially secure, have experienced stressful life events such as bereavement, and have negative beliefs about menopause are more likely to be depressed. In a recent study it was found that depression is also more frequent in women who have had a hysterectomy.[3] Expectations influence the experience too. Women who have the expectation that menopause will bring a host of physical and emotional problems are known to be more adversely affected by it.[4, 5, 6]

The 1988 survey of 445 Christchurch women ranging in ages from 35 to 60 years showed that women who have had a history of severe PMS and who lead a home-based lifestyle, spend much of their time doing housework and watching TV, and do not have a very emotionally satisfying living situation, tend to have a lot of the following symptoms: tiredness, tenseness, depression, crying spells, loss of interest, headaches, and pressure feelings in the head.[7]

Gail Sheehy writes: 'The greatest majority of the unhappiest women over 45 wish they could make a career change but feel they can't. Many designate their career as homemaker. Others have low-paying, dead-end jobs. They feel trapped by financial instability or preoccupied by family problems.'[8]

On the other hand, women who have a good sense of self-esteem, and feel generally optimistic about the future tend to take a greater interest in their health and longevity, and actively seek information and help with menopause.

A recent German study found that women with good body image and self-esteem who exercise regularly have few if any menopause symptoms. It also found that women with low self-esteem and a poor sense of their physical attractiveness who tended to identify with the traditional female role were less sexually active and had pronounced to extreme hot flushes and emotional symptoms at menopause.[9]

Another German study concludes that the factors most influencing the menopausal experience are cultural, level of education, work and social status, health, and self-image.[10]

WHAT IS MENOPAUSE AND HOW LONG WILL IT LAST?

Menopause literally means 'last period'. So it is something you don't know you've reached until about a year has gone by since you last menstruated. The common term given to the years leading up to the last period is peri-menopause and applies to the four or five years leading up to the last period and a year or so after. If a woman is going to have discomfort with menopause these will be the years when it is most likely to occur — the years before menopause.

The average age for menopause in this country is 51.5 years. Women in their thirties can find themselves experiencing menopause, and women as late as 58 and 59 may still be menstruating regularly. The factors known to affect the timing of menopause are:

- Genetic — we tend to go through menopause at the same time that our mother did
- Hysterectomy — can bring on an earlier menopause
- Tubal ligation
- Smoking
- Ovarian surgery
- Cancer drugs (chemotherapy)
- Sudden grief or shock

Factors that do not affect the timing are:
- Age of first period
- Timing of pregnancy, number of children
- No pregnancy
- The oral contraceptive pill

MENOPAUSE IS NOT A DISEASE!

First and foremost, menopause is *not* an illness. It is a normal life event which can bring difficulties only if there is some imbalance in physiology or psychology. Most menopause-related problems are due to wrong eating, lifestyle imbalances, including a lack of exercise, smoking, excessive alcohol consumption, stress and worry, and exposure to environmental chemicals.

Menopause is a transition. It is a time when the body adjusts to a new level of hormonal balance following the cessation of menstruation and the associated monthly production of the hormones oestrogen and progesterone. The ebb and flow of these hormones in the body has been regular and predictable since puberty. They have clear reproductive functions in building and preparing the uterine lining for successful implantation of the fertilised ovum. They also have a myriad of functions throughout the body that are unrelated to child-bearing. The extent of the roles of oestrogen and progesterone is far from understood but they are believed to be involved in at least 300 bodily processes. It is known that they influence bone re-building, brain function, the cardiovascular system, our skin, hair, and joints.

The hypothalamus in the brain, which normally coordinates so many of the body's functions with exquisite precision, isn't quite able to manage its usual balance. This can play havoc with sleeping patterns, body temperature, libido, mood, menstrual cycles and appetite, leaving you feeling estranged from your body.

When we reach menopause we may have been cruising along for years feeling reasonably OK and unaware that we weren't perfectly healthy. But irregularities and imbalances become apparent when the body is required to muster its resources to cope with suddenly fluctuating levels of hormones.

Menopause is a valuable marker of where we are at, and is a great opportunity to re-assess every aspect of our life and begin to make choices and decisions that will impact on us positively for the rest of our lives.

A WIDE RANGE OF TREATMENT OPTIONS

Women who do suffer uncomfortable symptoms at menopause can take heart. There are many steps you can take to relieve them. Most often dietary and lifestyle adjustments will be sufficient and, if not, there is a wealth of options in the form of traditional herbal treatments and natural therapies that effectively ease the transition.

It is well documented that the absence of menopausal discomfort for Asian women is linked to their diet, lifestyle, and use of traditional herbal medicines. Typically Asian diets are low in fat and rich in minerals, digestive fibre, antioxidants and plant hormones or phytoestrogens. Asian women report few if any hot flushes, and in Korea, the main symptom of menopause is joint pain in the hand![11] Asian women are also much less at risk for the post-menopausal diseases of breast cancer, heart disease and osteoporosis. Since 1983 there has been a revival of the traditional Kampo (herbal) medicines in Japan. Seventy per cent of Japanese gynaecologists now prescribe these to women at mid-life in preference to hormone replacement therapy.[12]

HORMONE REPLACEMENT THERAPY

Modern medicine offers treatment for menopause in the form of hormone replacement therapy (HRT). It masks the passage through menopause, and has been found to relieve hot flushes and night sweats, and can be effective in restoring vaginal tissue. But HRT is a controversial treatment. It has risks associated with long-term use, and it may bring side-effects like breast tenderness, leg cramps, bloating, weight gain, depression and headaches.

HRT is commonly prescribed to women who are at risk for osteoporosis and heart disease. It is internationally agreed that it can help slow down bone density loss, and it can reduce the risk of hip fractures in women currently or recently using it. However, its application in the prevention of heart disease is now in doubt and most informed doctors no longer recommend it. A very recent clinical trial examining the role of HRT in treating women with established heart disease reveals that it increases the risk of fatal heart attacks in the first year of use.[13]

We now know that HRT is not safe to be used long term — i.e., five or more years. Besides its potential for increasing the incidence of endometrial cancer, gall bladder disease and blood clots, HRT increases the risk of breast cancer after five years of use. Women who have used HRT for an average of 11 years have an increased risk of breast cancer of 35 per cent compared to women who have never used HRT. Although this translates into a small increase in numbers of women with the disease, it is nevertheless significant. The risk becomes greater as you age.[14, 15, 16]

Menopause is not a disease, yet many well women are taking these pharmaceuticals to treat hormone-related discomfort that may well respond to simple lifestyle and dietary changes. Well-meaning doctors are over-prescribing HRT to women at mid-life, often unaware that in many cases there are effective simpler alternatives.

We are the first generation to have artificially controlled our fertility through the use of synthetic hormones, and now we can further control the subtle orchestration of nature by applying the same synthetic hormones at mid-life. We must question the effect all these hormones (including the environmental oestrogen-mimicking hormones) are having on our health. It raises concerns when we acknowledge the alarming rise in serious reproductive disorders in Western countries — not least the dramatic increase in the incidence of breast cancer.

One can be forgiven for noting with some cynicism the vast profits this treatment brings the pharmaceutical companies. Providing a subsidy on HRT prescriptions to New Zealand women cost the government's Health Funding Authority $8,425,533 in 1997. The cost in 1993 was $6,674,144.

For women who would like the benefits of HRT without the risks and side-effects, supplementation with naturally occurring plant hormones, or 'nature-identical' hormones may be worth considering. These are discussed fully in Chapters 5 and 8.

Just as menopause is not a disease, being post-menopausal does not mean we are in a hormone-deficient state requiring replacement. It is a natural process, and the body achieves a new balance post-menopausally by producing hormones from the adrenal glands, the brain, muscles and hair follicles as well as continuing to produce lesser amounts of hormones from the ovaries.

Despite the lack of available information on alternatives from most medical practitioners, women do have a wide range of risk-free choices at menopause. Our challenge is to ease the passage through menopause and to educate ourselves about our physical requirements in order to achieve a health status that ensures us a long and fulfilling life.

3
ANCIENT WISDOM IN A MODERN WORLD

As humans we are inextricably connected to nature and the environment. We are as much a part of the body of nature as a tree or a hermit crab, but our modern lifestyles can cause us to forget it. We have the idea that we can live in isolation from nature, even seek to modify and control it — a concept that has repercussions now coming back to haunt us, with global warming and pollution threatening our very survival. We strive to have mastery over the laws of nature by harnessing atomic energy, manipulating DNA, even cloning ourselves, but ultimately we are part of the vast body of nature and dependent on it for our existence. By accepting this and working to live in accord with the laws and rhythms of nature, instead of opposing them, our environment and our bodies will be healthy. It is vital that we understand our connection to nature on an individual level, and it is critical for the survival of the planet as well.

Our bodies remind us of our connection to nature through the rhythms of our menstrual cycle and its relationship to the lunar cycle. We are conscious of the fundamental laws of day and night, of balanced rest and activity, and the unpleasant effects of ignoring them. Our bodies are designed to rest when the natural world does, and activity is naturally supported during daylight hours when the sun warms the atmosphere and our metabolism is geared for action. If we reverse this natural order and repeatedly stay up late and sleep by day, we will get sick. From season to season too we need to adjust our diet and lifestyle to be aligned with weather and temperature changes. The laws of nature that we see operating outside ourselves also operate within us. Ultimately we are nature!

Not surprisingly, recent research has found that we heal more quickly and efficiently when we connect to nature in even the most basic ways. In a study of patients recovering from surgery, researchers found that those who recuperated in a room within sight of a small grove of trees recovered more quickly than those unfortunate individuals who were only given the option of facing a brick wall.[1]

We may believe on an intellectual level that we are isolated from nature, but in reality we cannot be. Once we reach mid-life we are forced to accept that we are a part of nature and we must operate within nature's simple laws to sustain good health. Failure to adapt simply means that we get sick, because our bodies can no longer tolerate lack of exercise, inadequate diet, insufficient rest and a stressful lifestyle. If we have lived a life entirely in accord with laws of nature then at menopause (or at any time) we will be well. But our lack of self-care and the influence of a de-mineralised, chemically controlled environment means the reverse is often the case.

We need a system of medicine that will teach us how to live in accord with the laws of nature which govern the healthy functioning of the mind and body; a system that understands the basis of any disorder in terms of all the possible mind–body–environment interactions. Medicine as we know it treats us in pieces — it treats a symptom without taking our underlying health and lifestyle into account. It may temporarily relieve a problem, but without treating the cause, eventually another will appear to replace it.

44 MID-LIFE ENERGY & HAPPINESS

Ancient eastern systems of health have long recognised the body's innate ability to heal itself when treated in terms of its wholeness and relationship to the environment. These systems of health recognise the effects of the seasons, of day and night, and the bountiful healing properties of nature. Throughout Asia ancient traditional wisdom provides knowledge of treatments and lifestyle adjustments that bring the body back into balance through the use of diet and herbal applications, massage, acupuncture, yoga postures, martial arts and meditation.

T'ai Chi, for example, is a form of Chinese martial art that is very popular in Asia — especially among older people. It is usually performed outside and uses subtle movements that cause energy to flow in the body. T'ai Chi, according to traditional Chinese medicine, is an excellent way of accumulating energy (chi), storing it, and then circulating it through the body in order to balance it and prevent or heal disease. Studies show that T'ai Chi can improve strength, flexibility, and endurance in patients suffering from osteoarthritis, and that it is an excellent weight-bearing exercise which can decrease joint swelling and tenderness, improve balance, and reduce the incidence of falls in men and women over 70 years.[2] Other research has found T'ai Chi to be beneficial for heart disease, hypertension, substance-abuse disorders, and stress-related illnesses. T'ai Chi has been found especially useful as part of rehabilitation programmes for heart attack victims and patients suffering from rheumatoid arthritis.[3]

Interest in these ancient traditions is growing as we become more aware of the limitations of the Western medical model. We have much to gain from systems of health that have stood the test of time and may provide answers to some of the disorders of the late twentieth century that cannot be cured by surgery or medication.

Ayur Veda is the classical system of health from India, which comes from the ancient Vedic tradition. Ayur-Veda literally means 'science of life'. It is known as the 'mother' of all medicines because it pre-dates and has directly influenced Chinese, Ancient Greek, Western, and holistic medicine in general. It is a complete system

ANCIENT WISDOM IN A MODERN WORLD

of health that enables you to recognise that your physical well-being resides not only within your body, mind and emotions, but is fully connected to the biological cycles of nature, to the seasons, even to the deepest universal laws of nature.

Ayur-Veda has extensive documentation from 5000 years ago. Remarkably these records show medical understanding of advanced surgical techniques and knowledge of aspects of human physiology, like the circulatory system, only fully understood by modern medicine in this century. Traditional knowledge of the healing properties of plants provides treatments and antidotes for every disease. For example, many studies of an ancient Ayur-Vedic formula of fruits and herbs called Amrit Kalash have revealed it to be an antioxidant that is literally one thousand times more effective than vitamin E or vitamin C.[4]

Although Ayur-Veda is still practised in India, aspects that had been lost or limited through the influence of time (much of it lost during the British colonial rule) have been revived in the last 20 years. Ayur-Veda is now available to most Westerners and continues to increase in popularity as its benefits and immense practicality become known.*

Based on the laws of nature that govern the rhythms of life (for example, the seasons, day and night), Ayur-Veda is tuned to the individual and applies a range of simple treatments to create health and prevent disease. It encompasses the healing of body, mind and emotions through meditation, diet, lifestyle and rejuvenation

---

* In the early 1980s, the preeminent Indian scholar, founder of Transcendental Meditation, and teacher of the Vedic tradition, Maharishi Mahesh Yogi, gathered together many of the most knowledgeable and distinguished Indian physicians, Western physicians, researchers and scientists with the aim of restoring the ancient theory and practice of Ayur-Veda to the world after centuries of neglect. Since that time the Ayur-Vedic healing prescriptions and ancient techniques have been revived in full in their original precision and integrity and made available in Western countries. (This reformulation of Ayur-Veda is known as Maharishi's Vedic Approach to Health.)

techniques along with cleansing programmes and herbal treatments. All aspects of lifestyle are taken into consideration including exercise habits and even suitability of career choice. It is primarily a prevention-based system of health which recommends that individually tailored lifestyle, diet and stress management changes are adopted to create a balanced and healthy person. It is not simply a system of prevention or cure. It is a system designed to allow us to develop as individuals and evolve to realise the full potential of our mind, body and emotions. It offers the potential for good health to become perfect health.

Each of us is unique. We are born with a body type or constitution all our own that determines who we are, and also what our strengths and weaknesses are. Ayur-Veda uses precise and subtle techniques to determine constitutional characteristics and to diagnose disorders. The most commonly used is pulse diagnosis which when applied can accurately determine what particular body type the person has, and where imbalances or diseases are located. Our bodies give us signals that tell us what they need. Ayur-Veda teaches us how to recognise and respond to these signals.

Treatments range from precisely orchestrated purification and massage therapies called 'panchakarma' to herbal compounds, aroma therapy, music therapy, yoga postures and deep meditation. Daily diet is important and equally so the amount of food consumed and the times of eating.

Ayur-Veda brings the body more in tune with natural rhythms by applying many simple common-sense recommendations of the kind our grandmother used to tell us about, for example, having a daily routine and going to bed on time — being asleep by 10 o'clock and up at dawn. That simple principle coupled with having your main meal in the middle of the day when your digestive fire (like the sun's heat) is strongest can make a profound difference to your overall well-being.

Ayur-Veda is a non-invasive personalised system of health. It has an emphasis on rejuvenation therapies and is based on the fundamental principle that nature provides an antidote or

ANCIENT WISDOM IN A MODERN WORLD

balancing factor for any imbalance that may occur. Best of all, while its treatments often have side-benefits, it is completely lacking the side-effects that come with drugs and surgery.

AYUR-VEDA, WOMEN AND BODY TYPES

Ayur-Veda classifies the entire complex universe into just three groups: movements, energy transformations, and physical matter. There are three corresponding governing principles, called 'doshas'. Vata dosha is responsible for all movements in space and is described as having the qualities of the wind. Pitta dosha is responsible for all energy transformations including digestion and metabolism and has the qualities of fire. Kapha dosha is responsible for structure (solids and liquids) and has the quality of earth and water. Everything in nature can be classified according to the predominance of these doshas — music, food, plants, the seasons, even relationships!

What makes each of us unique is our own combination and proportions of Vata, Pitta, and Kapha, which give us our own mind and body type. For example, the qualities of Vata (like the wind) are quick, light, changeable and dry. Do you know someone who is speedy, thin, and changeable and has either dry skin or a dry sense of humour? They have a Vata mind and body type. An intense, ambitious or fiery person, maybe with a red face and a big appetite, is a Pitta type, while a more solid, strong and calm person is a Kapha type. (You can conclude that summer is the Pitta season; ice-cream is a Kapha food; and a butterfly is a Vata animal.)

According to your body type, you are prone to particular dosha imbalances. This means a Vata person is more susceptible to low bodyweight or constipation (dry bowel), anxiety and insomnia, while a Pitta person is more susceptible to 'burning' complaints like skin rashes or acid stomach, and to having a hot temper. A Kapha person may be prone to depression, gain weight and catching heavy colds. Of course each of us has our own combinations of the three doshas. An Ayur-Vedic physician is adept at identifying both body type and type of imbalance, and can prescribe balancing treatments

VATA — CHANGEABLE

In the body, Vata's role is to do with the movements of digestion (peristalsis) and the entire processing of food. It is also associated with the mind, emotions, respiratory tract, circulation and organs of elimination as well as bones and sexual organs. People who are predominantly Vata tend to be thin, quick, unpredictable, enthusiastic, and talkative. A balanced Vata person is always infectiously happy, and energetic. She is also optimistic, cheerful and exhilarating. When Vata dosha is out of balance it manifests as over-activity in the nervous system and is experienced as emotional fear, anxiety, memory lapses or vagueness, fatigue, weight loss, and general dryness — in the bowels, joints, and skin. Vata governs the life force and is the leading dosha. Women who are predominantly Vata need to create balance in their life by getting sufficient rest, warmth and nourishment and, most importantly, establishing a routine in their everyday life.

PITTA — INTENSE

Pitta is the 'heat' element in the body and it metabolises food into energy and healthy body tissue. It is responsible for the digestive fire, and is associated with the hormonal system, heart, blood, liver, intestine and biochemical reactions such as those required to produce energy. When Pitta predominates, a person tends to be fiery — intense, with a sharp and creative mind, reddish colouring in the skin and hair, freckles, and a competitive streak. The balanced Pitta person is sharp and intelligent with good powers of concentration. She is also content, joyous and pleasant. Pitta is the body's cooking system and when Pitta is out of balance there is excessive heat and accompanying inflammations such as skin eruptions (boils), ulcers, indigestion, emotional irritability and a 'hot' temper. Ideally a Pitta type of person should strive to lead a moderate lifestyle and favour cooling activities.

KAPHA — RELAXED

The Kapha principle is responsible for the body's structure — the bones, tissues, strength, and lubrication. It is specifically related to mucus and fluid production and is most apparent in the lungs, stomach, lymphatic system, mouth and joints. Kapha types are solid and steady, even-tempered and calm with impressive endurance and a larger body size that tends to gain weight easily. They are affectionate, tolerant, forgiving, generous and serene. When Kapha is out of balance, the body tends to have an excess of fluids, a tendency to respiratory and sinus problems, obesity, tumours, mental and physical lethargy and procrastination. Kapha women may need to stir themselves to action. They respond well to vigorous exercise.

AYUR-VEDA AND MID-LIFE

Each season of the year reflects a predominance of one of the doshas. Summer and early autumn is Pitta time, autumn and winter is Vata, and spring is Kapha. Even the day is divided into periods when one of the doshas dominates. From 10 am to 2 pm is Pitta time (when the digestive fire is strongest), 2 pm to 6 pm is Vata time, and 6 pm to 10 pm is Kapha time. The same times apply through the night. Pitta time is 10 pm to 2 am — the best time for quality of sleep. Vata time is from 2 am to 6 am — the time you are most likely to wake and worry if Vata is out of balance, and 6 am to 10 am is Kapha time again. If you have had a restless night, you are sure to feel sleepy again around 6 am when Kapha's calming influence takes over. However, sleeping through Kapha time can leave you feeling heavy and dull. Waking with the freshness of Vata at 6 am is nature's (and therefore the body's) ideal.

In the same way, our life span is dominated by each of the doshas in turn as we progress through it. From childhood to early adulthood is Kapha time as we grow in physical size and strength. Adulthood through to mid-fifties is Pitta time, when we are focused on careers and achievements, and retirement years are Vata years, when we enjoy the more spiritual expansive values of Vata, away from the driving, focused, controlling values of Pitta. For this reason, as we age, our symptoms of imbalance are often likely to be those associated with Vata. It is usually Vata that requires pacifying or reducing as that becomes the tendency given the overall influence. For example, as we age we may become more forgetful, our hair may thin, and our skin may become drier and wrinkled. All these are signs of Vata. Ayur-Veda's Vata-pacifying therapies slow down the ageing process by restoring moisture, increasing deep rest, and reducing stress. This is done through diet, a regular rest and meditation routine, consistent exercise regimes, massage involving the use of fine oils like sesame oils, and daily routines which encourage the body to function smoothly.

At menopause many women are inclined to experience symptoms recognisable as imbalanced Vata. We talk about being forgetful, clumsy, anxious, light-headed, having itchy skin, vaginal dryness, overall skin dryness, and sleeplessness — particularly at two in the morning, which is when Vata is predominant. All of these are Vata symptoms. When looked at in the context of Ayur-Veda, the majority of the symptoms of menopause reflect Vata out of balance. Even hot flushes, which must obviously be associated with Pitta (being heat), are actually initiated by Vata imbalance because Vata is to do with movement — Vata fans the fire!

Vata symptoms of menopause
Anxiety
Mood swings
Memory loss
Loss of confidence
Feelings of light-headedness
Panic attacks
Heart palpitations
Sleeplessness
Restlessness
Headaches (some)
Vaginal dryness

Itchy, drying skin
Hair changes (thinning, drying)
Aching joints
Leg cramps
Dissatisfaction with relationships
Hot flushes

Pitta symptoms of menopause
Hot flushes
Night sweats
Heavy bleeding
Anger, irritability, frustration

Kapha symptoms of menopause
Weight gain
Bloating/fluid retention
Breast tenderness
Fibroids
Loneliness
Fatigue
Depression

AYUR-VEDIC STRATEGIES FOR A COMFORTABLE MENOPAUSE

The following are suggestions of interventions that can smooth difficulties at menopause. (It is a good idea to see an Ayur-Veda consultant for a complete personalised programme. See Resources, page 224.)

1. Practise a meditation or relaxation technique (like TM) daily — this reduces the toll that stress takes on the body and enables the body to fight the associated wear and tear.
2. Do what you love to do — engaging in purposeful and enjoyable activity enlivens the heart and mind, and makes you resistant to the negative effects of growing older.

3. Take enough rest. Go to bed early, rise early. If you can get to bed around 10 pm you will have better quality of sleep and feel less anxious or agitated.
4. Eat fresh fruits and vegetables, grains and legumes on a regular basis — where possible organic fresh foods, not processed or preserved.
5. Reduce or eliminate alcohol or caffeinated drinks — these are known to aggravate Vata.
6. Follow a Vata pacifying diet if you recognise that your experiences tally with those of a Vata imbalance. That is, favour nourishing, sweet, sour, heavy, unctuous (oily) warm foods like soup and rice, also yoghurt and fresh cheeses, olive oil and a little butter. Avoid pungent, bitter, astringent, light, dry, cold foods (see Ayur-Veda Recipes, page 201).
7. Eat your main meal in the middle of the day, eat lightly at night.
8. Exercise daily (but never strain) — walk, swim or bicycle and practise gentle yoga postures.
9. Give yourself a daily morning sesame oil massage called 'abhyanga' by gently massaging two to three tablespoons of warm refined sesame oil into the scalp, followed by the temples, neck, arms, chest, back, abdomen, legs and feet. Use palms and fingers to work the oil into the skin. Leave on for a few minutes before washing off in the shower. This helps to calm you and settle Vata, and is wonderful for the skin! Avoid on days when you are menstruating.
10. If still menstruating, rest more on these days.

AYUR-VEDA AND DIET

Great attention is given to diet and digestion in Ayur-Veda, with the main emphasis on restoring balance to the doshas. Typically, we treat a doshic imbalance by doing the opposite. For example, a

ANCIENT WISDOM IN A MODERN WORLD

Pitta type who is constitutionally 'hot' would be advised to follow a diet that is cooling. Hot spicy food would obviously serve to aggravate in this instance. But where a person is a more Vata body type, warm food with spices to taste will provide a balance. There are six tastes described in classical Ayur-Vedic texts: sweet, sour, salty, bitter, pungent, astringent. All six tastes should be present in every meal while we favour those that are balancing for us. When the six tastes are present the food satisfies, and cravings or the urge to 'snack' become a thing of the past.

Examples of foods in each category are:

Sweet: honey, sugar, milk, butter, rice, pasta, bread
Sour: yoghurt, cheese, sour fruits like lemon
Salty: salt
Pungent: hot, spicy foods, peppers, ginger
Bitter: leafy green vegetables, turmeric
Astringent: beans, lentils

Vata is balanced by sweet, salty and sour. Pitta is balanced by bitter, sweet and astringent. Kapha is balanced by pungent, bitter and astringent.

Food suggestions

1. Endeavour to eat food as close to 'natural' as possible. Eat whatever fresh fruits and vegetables are in season, and unprocessed foods, free of pesticides and additives. Avoid frozen, canned and re-heated leftovers.
2. It is best to favour warm foods, especially in winter. Avoid drinking iced foods and beverages with food because they actually chill the digestive fire essential for efficient enzyme function. Pitta types can eat more cool foods — especially in summer.
3. Reduce consumption of meat and fowl. Eat mostly grains, vegetables and fruit.
4. Enjoy freshly squeezed fruit and vegetable juices daily.

5. Avoid excessive amounts of fats, refined sugar, caffeine, alcohol and chocolate.
6. Eat a balanced diet that includes the six tastes.

Ayur-Vedic eating tips

1. Eat when you are hungry. Eating without hunger is a primary cause of discomfort, pain, disease and accelerated ageing. If we have hunger when we eat, it means that the body will be able to process the food we have consumed. Without hunger, food begins to decompose in the gut leading to a build-up of toxins which block the channels of circulation throughout the body. Rather than eating when you are not hungry, have a cup of plain hot water instead.
2. Have your main meal in the middle of the day, and eat a lighter meal in the evening. Digestion (Pitta) is strongest at midday and food will be utilised most efficiently at that time. Studies have shown that you can eat a certain number of calories early in the day and not gain weight, whereas the same food eaten in the evening is stored as fat.
3. Eat to about two-thirds of your stomach's capacity. This is approximately equal to the amount of food that fits into your two cupped hands.
4. Always sit down to eat.
5. Try not to work, read, watch TV or drive while you eat. Focus your attention on the eating/chewing process — your digestion will be better for it. (See Ayur-Veda Recipes, page 201.)

REJUVENATION THERAPIES

Ayur-Vedic rejuvenation programmes act by cleansing the body of accumulated impurities, which Ayur-Veda says is the basis of ageing and disease. Called 'panchakarma', the treatments range from sophisticated warm herbal massages to cleansing herbal steam baths and gentle purification procedures. The experience is profoundly relaxing and invigorating. Panchakarma is designed to loosen impurities in bodily tissues, then eliminate them from the body altogether. Treatment is individualised depending on your body type.

Essential oils
Essential oils can be added to your bath, to skin lotions, massage oils and shampoos. They can also be diffused from an oil burner or taken in food, teas, or douches.

1. **Essential Oils for Vata**
- Angelica: reduces anxiety
- Cedarwood: calming, comforting, stimulating to the mind
- Clary sage: rejuvenating, increases libido, antidepressant, relieves intestinal and uterine cramps
- Dhavana: reduces fear and anxiety, balances the immune system
- Ginger: has warming qualities
- Rose: regulates menstruation, helps with migraine, detoxifies the liver
- St John's wort: good for joint pain, anti-inflammatory, calming
- Sandalwood: helps insomnia, anxiety, low libido, is calming

2. **Essential Oils for Pitta**
- Clary sage, melissa balm and rose: reduces anger, frustration, fevers and vaginitis
- Lemon balm: for anger and excess sweating
- Lavender: calming, sedative, helpful with mood swings and high blood pressure
- Sandalwood: assists uterine disorders and cystitis, is harmonising and tissue-regenerating

3. Essential Oils for Kapha

- Juniper: reduces swelling and excess fluids
- Cypress: relieves sorrow and depression
- Bay: decongestant
- Clary sage: antidepressant, revitalising, aphrodisiac
- Sage: detoxifies, heats the body, cleanses; recommended for water retention
- Geranium: immune stimulating, firms, tightens tissues, mood elevating
- Orange: uplifting, warming, helpful in bladder and kidney disorders[5]

By protecting ourselves from damaging environmental influences and stress with meditation programmes, and by embracing the simple principles of Ayur-Veda and strengthening our immune system, we can cast a whole new outlook on the mid-life years and ageing. A healthy mind and body naturally favours positive emotions over negative ones, so we quite spontaneously feel happier and more fulfilled. According to the ancient wisdom of Ayur-Veda, when we function in this way, our bodies respond, rewarding us with a long, enlightened life.

Susan had recently immigrated to New Zealand from South Africa. Soon after settling in she developed uncomfortable signs of menopause and was not coping well. She was deeply tired but despite this couldn't sleep well at night. She regularly woke around two or three in the morning and couldn't get back to sleep until close to dawn. During the day she was tearful, and frequently overwhelmed by hot flushes. She tried taking HRT, but reacted badly to it. 'I had reached a point where I felt desperate, and my husband was despairing too. I decided to try Ayur-Veda at the suggestion of a friend. I had a full consultation with an Ayur-Veda consultant and was impressed with her abilities to take my pulse and accurately comment on my digestion, and even my state of mind! She recommended a daily routine that included a main meal in the middle of the day and several other personally tailored things to do. She said that this would reduce Vata, which she said was out of balance. I took herbal preparations specially formulated for menopause, and enrolled for a course of panchakarma. It was truly blissful — five consecutive days of massage and steam treatment that was deeply restful and subtle, after which I began sleeping soundly. I truly haven't looked back — I am coping so well now, and provided I don't overdo things and stick as much as possible to the routine I have been given, the hot flushes even stay away. The thing I love about Ayur-Veda is that it is completely personal, and it feels so right!'

4

WHAT HAVE THEY DONE TO OUR FOOD?

You may drive out Nature with a pitchfork, yet she will ever hurry back to triumph in stealth over your foolish contempt.
Horace (65–8 BC)

You are at the supermarket doing the weekly buy. You are loading up on foods that make your busy life a little easier. Foods like sweet biscuits, mayonnaise, pasta sauce, breads, sandwich spreads, coffee, ice cream. Plus you are stocking up on margarine or butter and the 'good' foods — fresh fruit and vegetables, breakfast cereal and yoghurt.

We think we understand about the evils of eating too much refined sugar and the wrong fats — but ultimately we have to feed ourselves and our families, so we do the best we can to eat well. Foods are pretty safe anyway — New Zealand has an overseeing food standards authority which limits the nasty additives and protects us from known toxins and carcinogens, doesn't it?

Well you would hope so, but the reality, shockingly, is no.

Many of the foods on our supermarket shelves are processed,

refined, chemically preserved, and have artificial flavours and colours added to them. In fact, these days it is really difficult to find foods that are whole and unadulterated. And labelling is far from adequate — we are not told what additives are toxic, carcinogenic, or potentially dangerous. In New Zealand it is estimated that a child will have consumed at least 3.4 kg of food additives by the age of five.

Take a closer look at what we think are the really healthy foods — the fresh and beautiful fruit and vegetables. The amount of pesticides used on vegetables and fruits, and agricultural products in both New Zealand and the United States is astounding. Strawberries and peaches routinely contain residues from seven different pesticides. Lettuce and apples may harbour as many as nine different pesticide residues and even flour often contains residues from six different pesticides. However, the winner in the pesticide residue contest is, without a doubt, celery, which in a recent test was found to contain measurable amounts of residues from 17 different pesticides! The health effects of exposure to multiple pesticides simultaneously are unknown and little effort is being made to evaluate them. As a matter of fact, many pesticides, especially older ones, have not been tested at all for their carcinogenic effects.[1]

Even more frightening, data from the New Zealand Ministry of Health Total Diet Survey 1990/91 clearly shows that young children consume more pesticide residues from food than any other age group. New Zealand children also consume far more pesticide residues than do American children. For example, the average daily intake of pirimiphos methyl (a known mutagen) was found to be 185 times higher among New Zealand children than among children living in the United States. Similarly, the intake of fenitrothion (a suspected mutagen) was found to be 423 times higher among New Zealand children![2]

Meanwhile, the World Health Organization (WHO) estimates that pesticides cause three million severe poisoning cases and 220,000 deaths every year throughout the world. Delegates to the recent World Food Summit were also told that most pesticides used on rice crops are useless. Dr Kong Luen Heong from the International Rice Research Institute in the Philippines told the Summit that 80 per cent of pesticides sprayed on rice are applied at the wrong time or used for the wrong pests. 'Production would remain the same if farmers did not use them,' he said.

The International Agricultural Research Group of the World Bank believes that spraying rice crops can do more harm than good. The human toll from using the sprays is extensive; many pesticides widely used in Asia have long been banned in Europe and North America as being too toxic to humans. It is encouraging that scientists at the International Rice Research Institute are now turning away from pesticide use and concentrating on techniques for using natural predators to attack the weeds and pests affecting rice crops.[3]

Many of the chemicals introduced into and now contaminating the environment are hormone disrupting and have been found to be seriously affecting wildlife populations including fertility levels in birds, fish, shellfish and mammals, as well as birth deformities and behavioural abnormalities. It is believed that these chemicals are responsible for ominously lowered fertility levels in humans. In their powerful and disturbing book *Our Stolen Future*, which reveals the full horror of the impact and the destructive potential of these chemicals, the authors warn that we have to find a better, safer, more clever way to meet basic human needs before it is too late. 'For the past century the commerce in cheap, abundant synthetic chemicals has shaped agriculture, industrial processes, economies and societies. . . . Nothing . . . will be more important to human well-being and survival than the wisdom to appreciate that however great our knowledge, our ignorance is also vast.'[1]

These man-made chemical products have repeatedly been hastily released into the market without caution or long-term testing. Previous tragic mistakes with thalidomide, tryptophan, DDT, contaminated cattle feed, etc are examples of novel products approved by scientists who lacked natural caution. We have learned a hard lesson most recently from 'mad cow disease' where the reassurances of politicians and scientists proved to be idle.

FOOD HISTORY THIS CENTURY

Despite the growth in understanding of human nutrition in the latter half of this century, there has been an unexpected and huge rise in the diseases of Western civilisation since the Second World War. Diseases like coronary heart disease, diabetes, gallstones, obesity, etc are being linked to the reduction of health-promoting micro-nutrient and fibre-rich foods in the diet as a result of over-refining and processing.

Our diet in the 1990s is far from natural — packaged into pre-cooked convenience food and fast food which has little or no nutritional value. Many New Zealand children consume vast quantities of 'junk' food and some rarely have a home-cooked meal or fresh vegetables. Some disadvantaged New Zealand children are reported to set off to school each day with only a bag of chips and a bottle of fizzy drink for their lunch. A two-litre bottle of Coca-Cola has $37^1/_2$ teaspoons of sugar in it! In the 1500s every man, woman and child in Europe consumed an average of 1 kg of sugar in a year. Now in Western countries it averages about 50 kg per person per year.

If we look to the food available to early humans we can get a pretty good idea of our dietary needs. They lived on whole grains, vegetables, raw leafy greens, pulses, nuts, seeds, fruit and berries. Once hunting became possible they added meat and fish as secondary sources of the same micro-nutrients.

During the war years in Britain a campaign was mounted by the government whereby the public were educated about the importance of nutrition. Everyone became familiar with energy-giving and body-building foods, together with the vital 'protective foods' which supplied essential vitamins and minerals. These were whole foods — fresh fruit and vegetables, grains, seeds and pulses and dairy products.

Sir Francis Avery Jones explains the evolution of the understanding of human nutrition this century in his 1992 lecture published in the *Journal of Nutritional Medicine*: 'They were probably the only years in the twentieth century when the entire population [in Britain] young and old and especially the vulnerable groups, had the probability of achieving a near optimum intake of the known vitamins and other essential nutrients in addition to having sufficient protein and energy foods. Within a year of the start of the campaign by the Ministry of Food, the mortality rate began to fall in all age groups. The remarkable reduction in mortality by 1942 occurring so quickly and so uniformly at all ages may best be explained by the increased intake of protective nutrients, particularly vitamin C, tipping the scales in favour of survival when medical crises like pneumonia or surgical operations occurred.'

Unfortunately, nutritional education did not continue after the war and, after rationing ceased, the public increased their consumption of fats and took no time in returning to their white bread and sugary rich diet. 'Gradually it was realised over the next two decades that new health problems were emerging, with the unexpected increase in a number of disparate but seemingly diet-related conditions. These included coronary heart disease, hypertension, diabetes, dental caries, peptic ulcer, diverticular disease, gallstones, obesity, cancer in certain sites including the colon, pancreas and breast, constipation and haemorrhoids.'

ENTER, THE CHEMICALS

'Provided their accustomed food supply is available, animals and birds in the wild remain in good health, but once their natural environment is changed, they may become subject to diseases that seldom if ever occur in their fully natural state.'[5]

In the last 50 years the application of pesticides and herbicides by farmers to increase crop yields has abruptly added an ominous element to most of our foods. Life has evolved over millions of years, and adaptation to changes in the food supply have been

WHAT HAVE THEY DONE TO OUR FOOD? 63

infinitesimal and slow. New hazards in the environment require nature to develop a defence to protect itself. Only very slowly the human gut establishes a new interaction with a chemical in food, with unpredictable outcomes.

Now new viruses and diseases that baffle medical science are emerging. Human activity is changing the earth's climate. Initial studies now link pesticides like DDT and petrochemical pollutants (PCBs) to myriad effects including low sperm counts, genital deformities, infertility, hormonally triggered cancers such as breast and prostate, and neurological disorders in children such as hyperactivity and deficits in attention. Breast cancer, the most common cause of death among women aged 40–50, is on the increase.

THE FINAL STRAW

Now, as we enjoy the last days of the twentieth century, a new and far more serious development in food modification has taken place — genetic engineering. It is the next step on from the use of agricultural chemicals because its main purpose is to produce plants that will tolerate even higher levels of chemicals being sprayed on them. It is not a development that is in the interests of the food consumers. Experts predict that within ten years most of the food eaten globally will be genetically engineered.

Genetic engineering is an application of biotechnology (the name given to gene research) involving manipulation of the DNA strand and the transfer of genes between species in order to mimic certain desired characteristics. That means, for example, that some fish genes have been 'attached' to tomatoes, making the tomato slower to ripen, and that a petunia gene along with a cauliflower mosaic virus and a soil bacteria gene have been added to the soybean to make it resistant to a particular herbicide.

Genetic engineering is *not* the natural extension of natural breeding or natural selection. Where in nature do we find DNA from a fish, a scorpion, a spider, a virus, a bacterium, an animal, even a human introducing itself into the DNA of a vegetable?

Agriculture companies want to create plants that are better

in some way — ideally that will give them an edge over their competitors. If they are successful, the return for the company is enormous because if you can create a significantly different plant you can patent it. That means that the company will get a return on its investment every time a seed or plant of that variety is sold. These companies develop a package of goods. For example, they develop a plant to go with their herbicide or pesticide, or vice versa.

Crops currently targeted for genetically engineered tolerance to one or more herbicides include: alfalfa, canola (rapeseed), cotton, oats, petunia, potato, rice, sorghum, soybean, sugarbeet, sugarcane, sunflower, tobacco, tomato, wheat and others. It is clear that by creating crops resistant to its herbicides, a company can expand markets for its patented chemicals.

Dr Joseph Cummins, Professor Emeritus of Genetics at the University of Western Ontario, warns: 'Probably the greatest threat from genetically altered crops is the insertion of modified virus and insect virus genes into crops. It has been shown in the laboratory that genetic recombination will create highly virulent new viruses from such constructions. Certainly the widely used cauliflower mosaic virus is a potentially dangerous gene. It is a pararetrovirus meaning that it multiplies by making DNA from RNA messages. It is very similar to the Hepatitis B virus and related to HIV. Modified viruses could cause famine by destroying crops or cause human and animal diseases of tremendous power.'

Austria and Luxembourg rigidly oppose the importation of genetically modified organisms (GMOs). In Europe and the United Kingdom compulsory labelling of most foods that are genetically engineered (GE) or have GE ingredients has been instituted. In the UK, two large supermarket chains are banning GE products in their own labels, and a third is labelling all foods that have GE ingredients. A recent survey revealed that 61 per cent of Britons regard genetically modified (GM) food as unacceptable and 77 per cent support a ban on the commercial growing of GM crops until more is known about health risks and environmental impact. MPs in the House of Commons have even banned the use of GM food in their restaurants! Meanwhile the European Parliament Environmental Committee has called for an immediate moratorium on the approval of all new genetically modified products. In Australia and New Zealand, genetically engineered food is on our supermarket shelves but the public is largely uninformed about its application or its availability.

The Australia New Zealand Food Authority (ANZFA) made its decision in December 1998 that the majority of genetically altered foods to be sold in New Zealand will be labelled. Although it might be argued that there is no harm in allowing genetically engineered foods onto the market as people will have the choice to buy them or not, it could become harder and harder to detect all foods derived from genetically engineered sources. It is estimated that over 60 per cent of processed foods on the supermarket shelves contain components sourced from genetically engineered products. As more and more foods become modified in this way it is likely this 60 per cent will rise so high that people will have difficulty avoiding them even if they are labelled.

What can you do? Eat organic foods and keep abreast of developments. Read Sue Kedgley's book *Eating Safely in a Toxic World*, (Penguin, 1998). Learn to read food labels. Write to the Ministry of Health and Consumer Affairs and your local MP and demand that food not be tampered with. Write to your supermarket and ask them to provide you with GMO-free/organic food and, as a minimum, full labelling. Don't let this continue. Remember, it is purely an economic decision, one that at this time supports New Zealand's world trade obligations. There is no benefit whatsoever to the consumer.

Dr Margaret Mellon, Director of Agriculture & Biotechnology for the Union of Concerned Scientists, cautioned that agricultural biotechnology is 'not a miracle technology. It's had lots of mistakes. It's an expensive technology that's problematic.' She added that there are 'alternatives to biotechnology for feeding the world and achieving a truly sustainable agriculture, which are worthy goals, but the hype of biotechnology is obscuring the path'.

Back to the supermarket trolley. What can you eat? Sixty per cent of our processed food includes soy. If you want to avoid eating genetically engineered soy, you will need to steer clear of: margarine, cakes, icecream, baby food, pizza bases, instant milk drinks, tofu, soymilk, crackers, pasta, noodles, sausages, mayonnaise, sauces, seasoning, breakfast cereal, sweet biscuits, to name a few.

In reality you will probably have to shop around a bit. Find a store that sells organic food, and be meticulous in reading labels. There are good shops (in the cities anyway) that sell organic flours, coffee and tea, virtually everything. In Auckland there are organic fruit and vegetable coops and companies who will deliver to your door. Start growing your own.

ASPARTAME (NUTRASWEET)

Aspartame was discovered as a drug in the sixties. It is produced by combining two amino acids (phenylalanine and aspartic acid) and methanol (10 per cent wood alcohol). At temperatures exceeding 85°F (body temperature is 98.6°F) the substance breaks down into formaldehyde, formic acid, and diketopiperazine (an agent known to cause brain tumours). Aspartame was first approved in 1974 and then withdrawn because it was found to cause brain tumors in rats. However, it was approved again, over the objections of many scientists, in 1981. Fresh doubts have emerged recently with the publication of a paper focusing on the possibility that aspartame may be contributing to the increased incidence of brain cancer.[6] The researchers found that the introduction of aspartame into the USA in 1981 and into dry goods and soft drinks in 1983 was followed by an abrupt increase (1310 cases per year, approximately 10 per cent) of brain tumours.

Aspartame is found in virtually all products that are labelled 'diet'. The dominant producer of aspartame is the NutraSweet corporation and it is estimated that world sales are well in excess of $1000 million annually.

WHAT HAVE THEY DONE TO OUR FOOD? 67

Eighty per cent of all complaints volunteered to the Food and Drug Administration (FDA) in the US concern aspartame. More than 1000 calls have been received from airline pilots, who are heavy consumers of diet sodas, packets of 'blue sugar' and chewing gums. Many doctors have reported drastic improvement or disappearance of symptoms after removing aspartame from the patient's diet. On resumption, the symptoms tend to return. Symptoms reported to the FDA include: headache, nausea, vertigo, insomnia, numbness, blurred vision, blindness, memory loss, suicidal depression, personality and behaviour changes, hyperactivity, gastrointestinal disorders, seizures, skin lesions, muscle cramping and joint pain, fatigue, heart attack symptoms, hearing loss and tinnitus, pulmonary and cerebral oedemas, shock and death.

Eat:
- All organic foods (at this time not allowed to be genetically engineered)
- Whole foods: a wide range of fruit and vegetables, pulses, whole grains, nuts and seeds
- Lean or white meats or fish if required — avoid heavy meat protein
- Monounsaturated fats (olive oil), cold-pressed fresh polyunsaturated fats, small servings of saturated fats (butter, other animal fats)
- Whole raw, natural sugars

Avoid:
- Processed foods and chemical additives
- Flavour enhancers, colours
- Excessively processed fats and sugars
- Excess alcohol
- Artificial sweeteners (NutraSweet etc)
- Pesticide residues
- Genetically modified food

UNDERSTANDING THE FATS ISSUE

There is great confusion surrounding this subject. Authorities tell us that the primary cause of heart disease in New Zealand is our consumption of butter and that we should therefore all eat margarine. It is true that New Zealanders have the reputation of consuming butter in lethal amounts, and must reduce to a minimal daily intake. But did you know that overall it is actually safer to eat butter than margarine? Another generally unknown fact is that most cooking oils (barring olive oil) are bad for you.

The body converts all food that is extra to its needs into body fat, whether that food is protein, carbohydrate or saturated fat. Therefore, if we are eating more food than the body needs (which the majority of people are), and adding saturated (butter or animal) fat to our food, it follows that our body becomes overloaded and lays down fat cells. We need very little if any saturated fat in our diet.

There are roughly two groups of fats — saturated and unsaturated.

SATURATED FATS

These fats are stable, inactive and virtually inert. They are found in meat, dairy produce and tropical oils like palm and coconut. They are easily identifiable because their consistency is hard at room temperature. Saturated fat is important to the body as a source of energy and as a way of protecting it against the effects of cold. Compared with the environmental needs of people in previous centuries our need for these fats is much less critical. We exercise less in general and have insulated and heated homes and workplaces. Instead of burning off fat we have too much of it for our physical needs and it accumulates.

All oils and fats in our diet are made out of molecules called fatty acids. A diet high in saturated fatty acids (with straight molecules that pack together to form rigid structures) will make cell membranes that are hard and incapable of functioning properly. Heart disease is the long-term effect of a diet too high in saturated fats.

WHAT HAVE THEY DONE TO OUR FOOD? 69

Cholesterol

Only animal fats contain cholesterol, but all saturated fats can generate higher cholesterol production by the liver. Increasing fibre intake and antioxidant vitamins such as C, E and beta-carotene can help reduce the harm done by saturated fats. Switching to vegetable protein will increase fibre and eliminate a source of cholesterol.

UNSATURATED FATS — STRUCTURAL FATS

These come in two forms, monounsaturated fats and polyunsaturated fats. Both are more biologically active than saturated fats and are able to take part in important biochemical changes in the body that produce energy, create hormones and help burn stored fats.

1. Monounsaturates are only found in olive oil, flax seed oil, and orange roughy fish oil. They are liquid at room temperature, but cloudy or solid when cooled. Monounsaturated fats fall into the category of storage fats, similar to saturated fats, but have an active role in the body too. They are most famous for their ability to improve the ratio of 'good' cholesterol (high density lipids or HDL) to 'bad' cholesterol (low density lipids or LDL). 'Good' cholesterol, HDL, plays a protective role by transporting fats in the blood to the liver for disposal into bile. 'Bad' cholesterol, on the other hand, tends to deposit fats on the arteries. Monounsaturated fats increase the HDL/LDL ratio by lowering the LDL without lowering the HDL. Mediterranean cultures famous for their lavish use of olive oil are remarkably free of heart disease and some forms of cancer even though they have a high total fat intake.[7]

2. Polyunsaturates are found in vegetables and their oils (corn, sunflower seeds, peanuts, etc) and in oily fish. They are essential to the body because it cannot make structural fats — they have to be obtained directly from our food. Unlike saturated fats they do not become hard at room temperature, but are liquid and stay so even

70 MID-LIFE ENERGY & HAPPINESS

if refrigerated. Polyunsaturated fats are needed to give cell walls (membranes) their flexibility and fluidity and for converting nutrients into energy. Their other major function is that they are precursors to prostaglandins — vital molecules known as 'communicators' in that they pass messages from cell to cell. Prostaglandins control the function of cells and also regulate the way in which important chemical reactions take place in the body.

Unfortunately, most polyunsaturates are not healthy once they have been isolated from the food they come in. Raw polyunsaturated oils rapidly become rancid and create toxic free radicals once they have been exposed to air. This is another reason to favour monounsaturated fats, as they have a more stable molecular structure and do not become rancid so quickly.

Polyunsaturates will lower cholesterol but do not lower the HDL/LDL ratio. Exercise and monounsaturated fats will achieve this. Therefore, a low overall fat intake is desirable with a focus on monounsaturated fats.

THE TRUTH ABOUT MARGARINE

Vegetable oil, in its raw state, is rich in the essential fatty acid linoleic acid. However, vegetables don't naturally produce a solid fat and most of the oils in processed foods are hydrogenated to make them solid. Hydrogenisation is a process that turns an unsaturated fat into a saturated one by adding extra hydrogen atoms to the fatty-acid chain. This turns an oil into a solid fat like margarine, and creates a new type of fatty acid called a 'trans' fatty acid, which competes with the true essential fatty acids to replace them in the tissues. Not one margarine on the market is healthy! Excess trans fatty acids damage arteries and cause heart disease and unnaturally high levels of cholesterol.

It is estimated that 30,000 Americans die annually from the effects of excess trans fatty acids in their diet. One of the most important steps to good health is to eliminate all trans fatty acids from the diet — basically margarine, potato chips, baked goods, and some sweets. Check the labels at the supermarket and avoid anything that contains hydrogenated vegetable oil or partially hydrogenated vegetable oil.

Apparently the sewerage pipes in London beneath fast-food outlets regularly become blocked when their walls build up a solid encrustation of the congealed 'vegetable fat' used for deep frying foods. The substance has to be manually removed with pick axes and is then trucked off to rural England to feed the pigs!

ALL FATS GO RANCID

Polyunsaturated oils in bottles are nearly always rancid, and depleted of nutrients. Refrigeration will delay but not prevent rancidity. Unfortunately we can't smell it — vegetable oils have to go many times more rancid than animal fats before we notice. These rancid, oxidised fats can damage arteries, have been implicated in increased rates of heart disease, and are cancer causing. Rancid oil creates oxidation in the body. The negative effects of oxidation are the reason antioxidants have become so popular.[8]

Left at room temperature, an opened bottle of cooking oil will go rancid almost immediately — often they are rancid before we purchase them. Again, olive oil triumphs. It has high levels of naturally occurring antioxidants, and is a stable, even re-useable cooking oil. Canola oil is also monounsaturated but it has a toxic ingredient that has to be removed and is under added suspicion as it is one of the seeds being genetically engineered.

Oils that go rancid most quickly are the polyunsaturated safflower, sunflower, and cottonseed oils, followed by soy and corn oils. Whole foods also turn rancid — in the following order: walnuts, pine nuts, sesame seeds, Brazil nuts, pecans and pumpkin seeds. Less likely to go rancid are almonds, peanuts, pistachios and cashews. Macadamias, being largely monounsaturated, are the least likely to go 'off'.

Buy fresh nuts or crack your own. Buy the extra virgin (green) olive oil, which still has most or all of its nutrients. Buy cold-pressed virgin polyunsaturated oils in small amounts in glass containers. Check the use-by date before you purchase, then refrigerate and use quickly.

Olive oil has a long history of being good for health. A study published in the *Journal of the National Cancer Institute* reports that olive oil lowers the risk of breast cancer. The study also found that women who ate the most vegetables and fruit had 48 per cent less breast cancer compared to the group who ate the least.[9]

In summary:

Be aware of the dangers of eating processed foods — particularly if they include hydrogenated oils or polyunsaturated fats, which are almost certain to have been processed in some way. Even if they haven't, chances are they will be rancid.

Overall, reduce your intake of fats and oils. We need such a small amount each day. Favour eating fresh vegetables, seeds and nuts. Substitute cold-pressed virgin olive oil for other oils (it is definitely worth the extra cost). Butter is OK in small amounts and certainly preferable to margarine unless eaten in excess. It is a stable saturated fat. Even better, use clarified butter which has had the salt and milk solid residues removed. In baking use olive oil, butter or coconut oil (unrefined).

ESSENTIAL FATTY ACIDS

There are two essential fatty acids, linoleic and alpha-linolenic acid, from which the body is able to make all the other polyunsaturated fatty acids. These two unsaturated fats help you burn body fat, and build energy; they also help your body manufacture important hormones. They are called essential because that is literally what they are — the body must find them in the daily diet.

Linoleic acid

Linoleic acids are known as n-6 (or Omega-6) fatty acids. The best sources of linoleic acid (LA) are leafy vegetables and their oils, nuts and seeds, and seed sprouts. Linoleic acid is converted in the body by an enzyme called the delta-6-desaturase enzyme into gamma-linolenic acid or GLA. We need GLA in order to produce prostaglandins. (Prostaglandins pass messages from cell to cell, control the function of cells and also regulate the way in which important chemical reactions take place in the body.)

The healthy human body can synthesize GLA from LA, but in some cases this essential synthesis is blocked or interfered with by excess cholesterol, saturated fats, monounsaturated fats, alcohol, zinc deficiencies, excess sugar, and common viral infections. So there is probably a large part of the population who do not convert LA to GLA efficiently. Since GLA is a crucial step in the synthesis of prostaglandins, a deficiency can have serious consequences.

Evening primrose oil is one of the few food sources known that will supply GLA to the body. Other sources are borage or starflower oil, blackcurrant seed oil, and oil of javanicus. There are differences between these in terms of GLA content and how efficiently they are absorbed by the body. Studies to date conclude that evening primrose oil, the most researched of them all, offers the surest source of GLA and its many benefits.

Supplemental sources of GLA have been found to benefit a number of serious health conditions — in particular PMS, migraine,[10] heart disease, diabetes,[11] and rheumatoid arthritis.[12] Preliminary studies indicate that GLA may reduce tumour cells,[13] and may be a critical factor in calcium metabolism and the treatment of osteoporosis.[14]

Alpha-linolenic acid

Alpha-linolenic acids are known as n-3 (or Omega-3) fatty acids and are found in pumpkin seeds, flaxseeds, soybeans, walnuts, as well as oil from fish such as wild salmon, mackerel, sardines and trout. Linolenic acid is converted into eicosapentanoic acid (EPA) and then on to docosahexanoic acid (DHA) which are highly important in mediating inflammation. Fish oils that are high in n-3 fatty acids have significant anti-inflammatory effects. A recent Australian study recommends that people with rheumatoid arthritis emphasise n-3 fatty acids in their diet over n-6 fatty acids

— i.e., they should eat more fish, n-3 rich seeds like flax-seed, and vegetables. The researchers comment that humans evolved on a diet that had a ratio of approximately 2:1 n-6 to n-3 fatty acids. Modern diets with a vast excess of n-6 fatty acids (i.e., high concentrations of vegetable oils, such as safflower, sunflower and corn oils, hydrogenated oils, etc) have a 25:1 ratio of n-6 to n-3 fatty acids.[15] There is evidence that a high intake of n-6 fatty acids may be responsible for asthma symptoms and that these may be reduced by supplementation with fish oils and other n-3 rich fatty acids.[16]

5
NATURAL PLANT HORMONES

Everything a man needs to maintain good health can be found in nature. The true task of science is to find those things.
Paracelsus, the father of pharmacology

For thousands of years, the use of plants for health purposes and disease prevention has been at the centre of society. In fact it is from the plants with healing properties that the active ingredients have been isolated and chemically modified to produce many of the modern pharmaceutical drugs. For example, aspirin is made from the active ingredient salacin from the bark of the white willow tree. Therapeutic application of the bark of the willow can be traced back more than 2000 years when Hippocrates recommended chewing on it to relieve pain and fever.

There is on-going debate over whether the full value of the active constituent is realised by isolating it. It is believed by many that the whole plant with its total intelligence and subtle synergism provides the full benefit. For example, while the foxglove flower contains poisonous digitalis, it also contains a protective component that causes vomiting.

Most of us are well aware of the nutritional value of whole foods in that they provide us with vitamins, minerals, essential fatty acids, carbohydrates, proteins and protective antioxidants. More recently scientific attention has been drawn to the presence and influence of hormones in plants. These hormones are not identical to those produced by the human body, but are often quite similar in structure and function. Named phytoestrogens initially in the 1940s because of the observed infertility (oestrus) of sheep who grazed on pastures rich in clover, they are found in a wide range of plants including vegetables, cereals and legumes. 'Phyto' is the Greek word for plant and means 'that which grows'.

Although only recently scientifically documented, knowledge of phytohormone-rich plants has been passed down via ancient texts, folklore and oral traditions. The pomegranate, for example, is associated with fertility; the Thai vine *Pueraria mirifica* is used as a rejuvenating tonic and an aphrodisiac; in the middle ages, European clergy believed that hops and the herb *Vitex agnus castus* lowered libido.[1] Linseed was cultivated by the ancient Babylonians and laws were passed to make sure the citizens ate it daily. Pliny (23–79 AD) wrote, 'The trees furnish medicines that promote urine and menstruation.'

WHAT ARE HORMONES?

Hormones are chemical messengers produced by glands in the body, for example, the adrenal and pituitary glands and the ovaries. They are secreted into the bloodstream and move about the body to reach target cells which have receptor sites on the surface. Acting a little like a key in a lock, when the right hormone reaches the 'right' target cell it will become accepted by the target cell and perform its function within the cell. In the case of the lining of the uterus, for example, the hormone oestrogen will re-build it. (Oestrogen is a proliferative hormone — its function is to do with growth and increase.)

Phytoestrogens are not as potent as 'real' hormones, but are of increasing interest because it is now known that they have a multitude of hormone-like properties that can be beneficial to women. There is growing evidence that regular consumption of fruits, vegetables, grains and legumes rich in plant hormones can positively influence a woman's health and hormone balance, particularly at menopause. In a way the title 'phytoestrogens' is misleading as these plant hormones are not oestrogens at all, but once metabolised by bacteria in the human gut are known to have both a weak oestrogenic and an anti-oestrogenic effect. They have been shown to inhibit the growth of cancer cells, making them strong candidates for a natural anti-cancer role. In addition, they are antioxidants and so actively assist in the war against free-radical cell damage; they are antimutagenic (help resist cell mutation), antihypertensive (help to lower blood pressure), anti-inflammatory, and antiproliferative.[2]

There is increasing evidence that a regular diet of phytoestrogens may decrease menopause symptoms, including hot flushes, help prevent osteoporosis, and offer a high level of protection against the development of cancers of the breast and colon. Further evidence indicates that they may reduce the incidence of heart disease and may prevent prostate cancer in men when supplementary doses are taken.[3, 4, 5, 6, 7, 8]

The traditional diets of approximately half the world's population contain moderate to high levels of phytoestrogens. In Asian cultures women traditionally have a diet that is low in fat, high in fibre and rich in a wide variety of fresh fruit and vegetables. It is reported that some women in Asia eat up to 200 different vegetables on a regular basis, whereas we eat something like 20! They also consume rice and soy products like miso (a salty soybean paste used in soups and other dishes), soybean chips, tempeh and tofu.

Asian women do not have the difficulties at menopause that Western women do — very few experience hot flushes (4 per cent compared to 85 per cent in New Zealand women) and they are not at risk for the post-menopausal diseases of osteoporosis, breast cancer, and cardiovascular disease that Western women are. In Japan the consumption of phytoestrogens is estimated to be approximately 200mg a day (compared with 5mg in the typical Western diet) and the incidence of hot flushes, hormone-related cancers and osteoporosis is reported to be one of the lowest in the world.[9, 10]

In further evidence that diet is the key, a study of Japanese women who had immigrated to the United States found that when Western-style diet and lifestyle were adopted, the incidence of oestrogen-dependent cancers like breast cancer increased.[11]

Researchers gauge the effect of diet on oestrogen levels by measuring the amount of oestrogen excreted in the urine. Women who have diets high in plant food excrete significantly more oestrogen in their urine. One study, for example, showed that Japanese women eating traditional diets had much higher levels of oestrogen in their urine compared with American and Finnish women.[12] Another study showed that women who did not eat meat or dairy products had higher levels of oestrogen in their urine than women who did.[13]

There are four main classes of phytoestrogens:
- Isoflavones, found in legumes such as soybeans, chickpeas, mung beans and red clover.
- Lignans, found in cereals and vegetables and seeds such as linseed and sesame seed.
- Coumestans, found in sprouts (particularly soy sprouts), fodder crops and alfalfa.
- Saponins, found in ginseng and the wild yam.

Isoflavones are found in greatest abundance in soy. The soybean is considered one of the sacred plants in China. It is eaten in many forms in Asia — as tofu, soy-pickled vegetables, tempeh, and miso.

Lignans are formed during digestion when intestinal bacteria break down certain compounds in rye, wheat, sesame seeds and linseed (flaxseed).

Coumestans are the most potent of the phytoestrogens, but are still a weak form of oestrogen in the body. The best source is from soybean sprouts and alfalfa sprouts.

Saponins are 'soapy' compounds which convert to sapogenins in the body. Some saponins can act weakly with oestrogen receptor sites like other phytoestrogens.

Based on this evidence, it is suggested that Western women could most effectively change their diet to include more of these foods. One way is to consume 30–50mg of soy products per day. This could be achieved by eating one serving of tofu (120 g) or two servings of soy milk (200 ml each), or four slices of soy-enriched bread.[14] Several women have reported a reduction in flushes when they have included soy milk in their diet. One woman who was not sleeping well and had experienced increased breast size at menopause ate tofu every day for three weeks and found that her breasts had returned to normal and she was sleeping well again. Health-food stores now offer soy as a powdered or tableted supplement which may be easier to take for some. At present most of the phytoestrogen research has been conducted on soy, even though there are many other excellent plant sources of phytoestrogens.

Phytoestrogens are known to be transformed by bacteria present in the intestine into active compounds in the bloodstream that have a weak oestrogenic effect.[15] In order to metabolise phytoestrogens successfully, therefore, certain bacteria must be present in the gut. It is possible that a lack of these could account for limited results for some women, and that the use of antibiotics could also reduce the effectiveness.

SOY IS CONTROVERSIAL

There have been warnings in New Zealand against feeding soy milk to infants, as large quantities of hormone, even weak plant hormone, may be inappropriate for children. However, in Asian countries there is no evidence of any adverse effects on children who eat these foods as their parents do. There is a lack of information on the effect of soy phytoestrogens on infants whose mothers normally consume a Western diet, and studies in this area are on-going.

Despite centuries of use in Asia, concerns have been raised that soy contains ingredients called protease inhibitors and phytates, which may affect the body's ability to absorb iron and other minerals. It is believed that most Western methods of processing and cooking don't eliminate these ingredients. Asian methods of preparation often involve fermentation and heating, which may have evolved as a way to break down the 'unwanted' ingredients. Some concerned researchers warn that manufacturers may be jumping the gun and marketing soy products before safety has been established.[16] Others report that these ingredients have good properties, and that when soybeans with high amounts of protease inhibitors were fed to animals there was a substantial reduction in experimentally induced breast cancer.[17] They also report that higher levels of phytates in the diet decreased the rate of cellular division in samples of breast tissue.[18]

Soy is also under suspicion because it is now being genetically engineered to be resistant to the herbicide 'Roundup'. These 'Roundup resistant' soybeans have been found to contain much higher levels of phytoestrogens. The effect of this and the altered genetic material on humans who consume them is unknown and untested. To avoid consuming genetically engineered soy, you must eat products labelled as organic. Some of the speciality soy and linseed breads available in New Zealand are reputed to be made from soy flour that is sourced from non-genetically engineered stock, as are the powdered soy supplements mentioned above. You may wish to check with the manufacturer.

Genetically engineered soy is also used as a bulk additive in processed foods, and it is estimated that about 60 per cent of foods, including margarine, cakes, icecream, pasta, pizza bases, biscuits, mayonnaise, etc, have added soy flour. If you want to by-pass these controversial and potentially hazardous products, it might be better to look to the many other, possibly safer, plant sources for your daily intake of phytoestrogens.

It is undoubtedly wise to include a wide range of vegetables in your diet and to include a variety of grains, legumes, fruits and seeds. Think about what people would have eaten in ancient civilisations — organic, freshly grown whole foods. Perhaps consider growing your own — it is a wonderful way to exercise, be creative and feed yourself and others life-giving food. Various New

Zealand seed companies now offer a great range of unusual and special vegetable seeds including very tasty Asian green vegetables. These are easy to grow, don't require a huge amount of effort, and can even be grown in containers. They are a rich source of vitamins and minerals. (See Resources, page 224)

Foods rich in plant hormone are:

- Legumes: soybeans, chickpeas, lentils, mung, haricot, broad, kidney and lima beans, and products of beans, such as soy grits, soy flour, tofu, and soy milk
- Wholegrain cereals: wheat, wheatgerm, barley, hops, rye, rice, bran, oats
- Fruit: cherries, apples, pears, stone fruits, rhubarb
- Seeds: linseed, sunflower, anise, sesame
- Vegetables: green and yellow vegetables including kumara, carrots, fennel, onion, garlic
- Vegetable oils: olive oil
- Ginseng, liquorice, hops
- Soy-linseed bread

PHYTOESTROGEN SUPPLEMENTS

There are a wealth of products on the market containing phyto-hormone-rich plants in the form of herbs, like red clover, and powdered soy, etc, which can be helpful at menopause. These appear to work really well for some women and not at all for others. Perhaps some of us have more of the required intestinal bacteria than others but it is certainly worth investigating what is available and giving them a try. It is best to try only one product at a time (so that you know what is working), and to keep to the stated dose. These compounds will offer a higher daily intake of phytoestrogen than you would normally get in your diet. In the main they are traditional medicinal herbs that have stood the test of time and are well documented for their effectiveness even if they haven't all been as well researched in controlled studies as orthodox treatments like HRT.

Concerns are regularly expressed about the safety of self-prescribed, over-the-counter treatments even though a recent poll of New Zealanders showed that 74 per cent of households use herbs, vitamins, minerals, and other natural products.[19] Few herbs approved for sale in New Zealand have side-effects or risks associated with them. If you buy well-known labels and take the correct dosage, you are unlikely to experience problems. It is a good idea to take products in divided doses throughout the day for maximum benefit. Most of the herbs listed below have a tonic effect, and once the benefit is felt can be gradually reduced without further problems.

If you are unsure, you could take the personally tailored advice of a herbalist or health practitioner.

BLACK COHOSH
Cimicifuga racemosa

A North American Indian plant, the root of black cohosh has a long tradition of use. The shamans of North American tribes and later the American colonists used black cohosh extracts for joint pain, myalgia, and neuralgia as well as for menopause symptoms, general female reproductive complaints, pain in childbirth (hence its common name 'squaw root') and rheumatism. A similar species, *Cimicifuga rhizoma*, has also been used similarly in traditional Chinese medicine.[20]

Until recently, black cohosh was believed to contain phytoestrogens. However, it is now known that it does not contain isoflavones, but it does still bind to oestrogen receptors. Because it appears to have no oestrogenic qualities, it is considered safe and suitable for use by women who have menopause symptoms like hot flushes and have a history of breast cancer.[21]

Black cohosh has been used extensively in Germany for the last 40 years, which accounts for it being the home of many clinical trials measuring its effectiveness. Recent studies have found that it is more effective than conjugated oestrogens (HRT) in reducing hot flushes and that in many cases women could be switched to it from HRT without problems and with equivalent success.[22]

Black cohosh is available as a dried herb or in combination with others especially blended for mid-life women. It will help to reduce the intensity and frequency of hot flushes. It is calming, and has been shown to be helpful for menopausal mood swings, anxiety and depression when combined with St John's wort.[23]

It should not be used to treat pregnant women or when there is menstrual flooding.

CHASTE TREE
Vitex agnus castus

A native to Southern Europe and Western Asia, the part used medicinally is the small blackish aromatic fruits or berries. It is also known as Monk's Pepper because it was given to medieval monks who were considered to be too lustful in their thinking![24] (It is reputed to have the opposite effect in women.)

This is a remarkable herb, first mentioned by Hippocrates in 450 BC: 'If blood flows from the womb, let the woman drink dark wine in which the leaves of the Vitex have been steeped.' The herb is also referred to in Homer's sixth century BC epic, the *Iliad*.

Chaste berries have been found to be effective in treating PMS, menopausal symptoms of hot flushing, dry vagina, dizziness and depression, and normalising irregular perimenopausal bleeding. They have been found to be helpful with acne and other skin problems and help to restore digestion. They also help reduce breast lumps and tenderness and restore emotional calm. The two most quoted studies are from Germany. Each trial included over 1500 women. Both patients and physicians reported 90 per cent relief from symptoms of PMS after one month.[25] In a similar study patients were followed for up to six years. In 90 per cent of women the chaste berry relieved their PMS symptoms.[26] The berries have been found to enhance progesterone and luteinising hormone. Good results can take time, but many women report excellent results after 8–12 weeks.

Precautions: Excess use may cause itching, rash, or nausea. Not recommended for use in pregnancy or while on HRT or other hormone treatment including oral contraceptives. (It has, however, been recommended for use when re-establishing balance after taking the oral contraceptive pill.) It is not recommended post-menopausally.

DONG QUAI/TANG KUEI
Angelica sinensis

The root stock of this plant is prescribed for almost every gynaecologic ailment except pregnancy or heavy menstrual bleeding. It has been used in China for centuries and is highly revered. Research has shown that it regulates the function of the heart and uterus.[27] It is excellent for treating hot flushes and will work quickly for many women. It does have a warming effect, however, so if you feel generally hot throughout the day it may not be for you. It will also relieve uterine cramps and revive thinning vaginal tissue. It is known to be calming and nourishing and helps with aching joints during and after menopause.

Precautions: Do not take if you have heavy menstrual bleeding as it relaxes the uterus. Avoid if you have fibroids.[28]

SAGE
Salvia officinalis

Salvia means 'saviour'. It has been used since ancient times by the Chinese, the Romans and the Native Americans. The essential oil in sage is antiseptic. It is most effective for relieving hot flushes and night sweats and, like black cohosh, can be as effective as HRT. According to Susun Weed in her book *The Menopausal Years*, 'there is no other herb so effective at drying up the flowing springs of perspiration that gush with some women's hot flushes'. She goes on to say that it will relieve dizziness, trembling, and emotional swings, ease irritated nerves, eliminate headaches, and aid digestion.[29]

Pick a bunch of sage from your garden and make an infusion by pouring over boiling water and letting it steep (or use dried sage — three teaspoons per litre). Draw off the liquid and drink one tablespoon of the mixture throughout the day, or try half a cup at bedtime to prevent night sweats.

GINSENG
Panax ginseng

Oriental ginseng has been used for pharmacological purposes for over 4000 years. It was traditionally used for the prevention and treatment of a wide number of diseases. According to the Shanghun lun written by Zhangji of the Han dynasty in China (circa 200 AD), ginseng was prescribed for headaches, lack of strength, fatigue, dizziness, nausea and vomiting, diarrhoea, asthma, uterine haemorrhage and impotence.[30] Leslie Kenton in her book *Passage to Power* notes: 'It has been praised for centuries for its rejuvenating properties, its ability to protect against illness, to enhance the body's ability to handle stress — even to prolong life. The herb is a great ally — the most potent of all the plants for handling very severe symptoms in menopausal women.'[31]

Ginseng will regulate hormones and stop menstrual flooding, reduce the intensity and frequency of hot flushes, enhance libido, and improve energy levels and digestion. Its rejuvenating effects are linked to its excellent antioxidant properties.

Always buy the best (probably the most expensive) form of ginseng for maximum effectiveness.

RED CLOVER
Trifolium pratense

Claimed to be nature's richest source of isoflavones, red clover has recently become available to women as an over-the-counter product. Introduced into New Zealand pharmacies and health food stores in February 1998 along with considerable advertising, 9000 packs were sold in the first three and a half weeks! A sure indicator of how much need there is for help with menopause.

Like other herbal treatments, the results can take a few weeks to manifest, but many women are reporting good results. After taking red clover for four months one woman experienced an improvement in her mood swings and depression, and was sleeping better at night. After only two weeks' use her bladder frequency had normalised and the night sweats had disappeared.

There is preliminary evidence that red clover may also help prevent and treat prostate cancer in men.[32]

Red clover can be taken in tablet form or drunk as an infusion made from the dried flower heads. To do this, quarter-fill a container with clover blossom and fill with boiling water. Place the lid on and leave for at least four hours to make a strong brew. Squeeze the plant material and discard. Drink ½ cup of the liquid at room temperature, two or three times daily, hot or cold. You may add mint to make it more pleasant tasting.

WILD YAM
Discorea villosa

The wild yam is not the yam that we grow in New Zealand. It is a large oily tuberous root vegetable which grows in the Pacific Islands and in Mexico. It has become the focus of much attention in recent years as it contains steroidal saponins which have both an oestrogenic and progesterone-like action in the body.

Although it has been used traditionally to prevent miscarriage and as a contraceptive in the Trobriand Islands, its uses in the West have to date been mainly pharmaceutical. The cultivated yam produces the hormone diosgenin, which pharmaceutical companies convert to the synthetic progesterone medroxyprogesterone, and oestrogens which are used in the oral contraceptive pill and in HRT.

It does, however, have effective properties as a herb and can be purchased as a powder, or as a cream which, especially when combined with other herbs such as sage, St John's wort and black cohosh, can help reduce hot flushes, depression and sweating. It also has anti-inflammatory properties and will help with joint and muscle pain. It stimulates libido in many women. There are no known side-effects.

For further information on herbs for menopause, read Leslie Kenton's *Passage to Power*, or Susun Weed's *Menopausal Years. The Wise Woman's Way*.

6
NATURAL HORMONE REPLACEMENT

The recent availability of a 'nature identical' type of hormone replacement offers women a promising alternative to the controversial synthetic hormone replacement therapy (HRT). Understandably the body can better tolerate the introduction of natural and identifiable hormones rather than synthetic ones which cannot interact in the same precise and appropriate way. For those women who opt for this type of treatment, natural hormone replacement appears to provide a better hormonal balance without unpleasant side-effects or health risks. Women of the post-war generation are notable for their interest in things 'natural', and many have a reluctance towards taking synthetic pharmaceutical treatments with known or unknown side-effects.

For the past year or two, New Zealand women have mostly been hearing about natural progesterone, usually in a cream form — from the internet, in books, from friends who have tried it. They have been able to access it either over the counter or from multi-level marketing distributors. Having tried it, their relief is often so rapid that enthusiasm has spread. It may not be the miracle cure

NATURAL HORMONE REPLACEMENT

for everyone, but for many women who are suffering from PMS and some of the harsher symptoms of menopause it appears to offer great relief. Many doctors are now confirming that their patients are showing positive results. In addition there is some evidence that progesterone may be an effective treatment for reversing bone density loss.

For many women, natural progesterone seems to provide the answer they are looking for. Mary's story is a common one: 'I had been travelling for a month in the US and had gone from our mid-winter to their summer. My hot flushes were unbearable, I wasn't sleeping at all well, and I ended up getting some sort of infection, probably because I was so run down. When I returned I started to use natural progesterone cream on the recommendation of a friend. The result was dramatic. I slept deeply and long the very first night after applying a small amount of the cream. It was a day or two before I realised that the hot flushes had fully disappeared. I couldn't believe it. I continue to use the cream with same result.'

WHAT IS IT EXACTLY?

As we have already seen, many plants contain hormones. These are sometimes similar in molecular structure to those produced in the body. In the case of natural progesterone, the plant hormone diosgenin from the wild yam is used as a precursor molecule. (Soya is also used for this purpose.) Diosgenin is converted to a product with the same molecular structure as the progesterone that is produced by the ovaries. It is a 'natural' hormone in that it is 'nature identical', but it is not found in plants in this form.

The progesterone components of hormones prescribed in standard HRT are called progestagens or progestins. It is important to understand that these are not nature identical and that when we refer to progesterone here we mean natural progesterone, not synthetic progesterone.

The intense interest in the use of natural hormones was initially generated from the work conducted by Dr Katherina Dalton in Great Britain. Dr Dalton published widely in medical literature between 1953 and 1983 and has 41 original papers to her credit. She has published articles and books on her use of natural progesterone in treating migraine and PMS.[1,2]

The New Zealand public are more aware of the work of Dr John Lee MD, who collaborated with scientist Dr Ray Peat in sourcing the research and publishing articles on the use of natural progesterone. Dr Lee worked for some 20 years with natural progesterone in his general practice. He has strongly influenced American public opinion and, since retiring from practice, his influence in this field has continued to grow as success and popularity with the therapy spreads.

The pioneering work of Dr John Lee has revealed the application of natural progesterone in treating PMS, symptoms of menopause, osteoporosis and other hormone-related female disorders like fibrocystic breasts and endometriosis. In his book *What Your Doctor May Not Tell You About Menopause* he says, 'I don't know of any reason why any woman should be subjected to synthetic hormones. The natural hormones are available and are much safer and freer of side effects.'[3]

There is not the same depth of published literature on this subject that there is on HRT. This is because natural hormones cannot be patented, and there has been little commercial backing for research, as is the case with many naturally occurring treatments. However, some studies have been done and many more are currently underway.

Research has indicated that natural progesterone may be a useful tool in the treatment of heart disease. A 1995 study measured the levels of HDL ('good') cholesterol in a group of 875 postmenopausal women given a range of synthetic and natural hormone replacement options or placebo. Even though it was taken in conjunction with oestrogen, the study brought results in favour of natural progesterone, which surprised the investigators. The prominent cardiology researcher Elizabeth Barrett-Connor, who was heading the study, reported that if women were worried about heart disease, she would consider prescribing them natural progesterone rather than progestagen.[4]

Progesterone also appears to have a protective role against breast cancer. A 30-year retrospective study at Johns Hopkins University found that women who were progesterone deficient had 5.4 times the incidence of breast cancer and there were a greater number of deaths from cancers of all kinds.[5] A double-blind randomised study has shown that progesterone actually slows the rate of cancer cell division in breast duct cells.[6] At a recent world conference on the menopause, European specialists advocated the use of progestins, which are as close as possible to natural progesterone, in the treatment of breast cancer. They predicted that this was a treatment we would hear more of in the future.[7]

PROGESTERONE AND BONE DENSITY INCREASE

There is initial evidence that progesterone has the ability to increase bone density. However, at this time no large clinical trials have been done to verify this. Dr John Lee used repeated bone density measurements on his patients and reported a remarkable average bone density increase of 10 per cent in the first six to twelve months with an annual increase thereafter of 3–5 per cent.[8] There has been some earlier published evidence that progesterone is a bone-building hormone.[9] This has prompted a study of 60 women, currently underway at the Chelsea & Westminster Hospital in London.

Several New Zealand women have reported increases in bone mineral density since using natural progesterone cream. In two recent examples, an 83-year-old woman was found to have established osteoporosis in both hip and spine after a DEXA scan (see page 120) in 1997. After exactly one year of treatment with natural progesterone her bone density had increased significantly. And a 50-year-old woman whose spine showed degenerative change in the direction of osteoporosis was similarly found to show significant improvement after one year's use of natural progesterone.

There is a wealth of anecdotal evidence that the application of natural progesterone, either as a cream or in an oral form, can reduce symptoms of:

- PMS — particularly cramping, fatigue, headaches, irritability, sleeplessness
- Menopause — hot flushes, lower libido, dry vagina, migraine, sleep disturbances.

WHY HAVE ANY HORMONE AT ALL?

Although more research is needed, there is logic behind replacing hormones to give physiological (normal) levels of progesterone in the pre- or peri-menopausal woman. Women with hormone-related disturbances are often told that what they are lacking is oestrogen. But looking at the typical pattern of menstrual activity in the years leading up to menopause it is clear that the hormone most likely to be lacking is progesterone. This fact seems obvious upon investigation but it seems to have eluded most medical practitioners under the bombardment of oestrogen-promoting material they receive from the pharmaceutical companies.

If we look at the fascinating cyclical rise and fall of reproductive hormones in the monthly female cycle and combine that with the evidence that women have fewer and fewer 'fertile' cycles in their late thirties and through their forties, it is obvious that we are producing much lower levels of progesterone while maintaining at least some production of oestrogen. In fact, we know that the ovaries continue to produce oestrogen after menopause — possibly up to 40 per cent of what they did before menopause.[10]

THE EXQUISITE PRECISION OF THE MONTHLY CYCLE

Consider the delicate orchestration of the monthly cycle. It is quite miraculous and well worth understanding. Through our fertile years there is a constant monthly rise and fall of the hormones oestrogen and progesterone. They have clearly defined reproductive functions, but they have additional influences and functions throughout the entire body. Since puberty our bodies have been accustomed to the regular monthly wash of reproductive hormones — delivered to the brain, bones, skin and cardiovascular system via the blood.

THE ROLE OF THE BRAIN

On day one of the menstrual cycle, the hypothalamus in the brain is triggered to produce a hormone known as gonadotrophin-releasing hormone (gnRH). This in turn stimulates the pituitary gland to produce the hormone follicle-stimulating hormone (FSH). The rise of FSH in the blood has the effect on the ovaries of encouraging between 15 and 20 egg cells to begin ripening in egg follicles. It is not understood why this number of egg follicles begin to ripen, or why one of them will grow more than the others and make its way to the surface of the ovary, but this is the scenario every month.

OVULATION

As the egg follicles ripen they begin to produce the hormone oestrogen. Oestrogen is responsible for rebuilding the lining of the uterus, which has been shed during menstruation, so as the egg follicles ripen and grow, and oestrogen levels correspondingly increase, the uterine lining re-builds. At about day 10 or 12, the oestrogen levels peak in the blood and a feedback mechanism to the brain is triggered. The hypothalamus responds to this high level of oestrogen by causing a change in the gonadotrophin-releasing hormone. The altered hormone stimulates the pituitary gland to produce another hormone — luteinising hormone (LH). The surge of LH in the bloodstream causes the egg follicle that has ripened the most to rupture and release the now mature egg cell. This is the process of ovulation.

The released egg cell (ovum) is wafted up into the Fallopian tube by the fronded finger-like ends, which are suspended over the ovaries. The responsibility of the ovary for the egg is now complete.

THE REMARKABLE CORPUS LUTEUM

The work of the egg follicle is not over, however. Having released the egg, the follicle collapses back on itself and forms an organ called the corpus luteum or 'yellow body'. ('Luteus' means yellow in Latin.) This new organ then produces the hormone progesterone, which begins to rise in the blood as the level of oestrogen begins to fall. Progesterone has the reproductive function of preparing the uterine lining for implantation should fertilisation of the ovum occur. This means that the lining doesn't grow any bigger, but glands in the uterus produce nutritious substances and create an environment conducive to sustaining pregnancy.

MENSTRUATION

After about 28 days, if fertilisation of the ovum has not taken place, then the levels of progesterone and oestrogen drop suddenly and the uterine lining is shed once more. This sudden drop of hormones is the trigger to the hypothalamus to again begin its production of gnRH.

It is miraculous. The study of the mechanics of conception is even more awe-inspiring but we will leave it there.

THE APPROACH TO MENOPAUSE

As we age, as early as our mid-thirties, we begin to have variations on the above pattern. Our ovaries start to respond differently — often more sluggishly — to the stimulation of the hypothalamus and the pituitary hormones and may not ripen the same number of egg follicles, or to the same degree. This can result in lower levels of oestrogen being produced, and the mid-month peak not being achieved to trigger the production of luteinising hormone. Without the production of LH, ovulation does not occur, and if ovulation doesn't occur, then the corpus luteum is not formed and progesterone is not produced. So in many cases, long before the ovaries cease to produce oestrogen, they could have ceased to produce progesterone. Our periods may appear to continue as normal or they may be lighter or heavier, but it is not obvious to us whether we ovulate or not.

TOO MUCH OESTROGEN?

The fact that so many women respond well to a natural progesterone replacement rather than oestrogen lends weight to the theory that our bodies often have more than enough oestrogen anyway. Modern life with its low-fibre, high-fat diet, and our exposure to environmental pollutants that are oestrogen mimicking creates, among other things, an imbalance of hormones. Add years of taking the oral contraceptive pill to that and many women may have had too much oestrogen and not enough progesterone for their entire reproductive lives. Dr Lee refers in his book to a state of 'oestrogen dominance' rather than oestrogen deficiency. Oestrogen dominance brings its own set of problems — namely weight gain, headaches, uterine cramping, sore breasts, bloating and heavy periods.

You may have more oestrogen than you need because:
- your diet is low in fibre and high in fat, which reduces the excretion of unwanted oestrogen in the stool;
- you are not ovulating regularly but your ovaries are still producing quite high levels of oestrogen;
- you have been taking the contraceptive pill or oestrogen replacement;
- you have been exposed to environmental oestrogens.

WHAT ARE ENVIRONMENTAL OESTROGENS?

This is a disturbing global issue, which again reflects the effect of man's unchecked use of chemicals in the last 50 years. It is another sign, along with global warming, that our efforts to control the environment have backfired badly, and the environment is retaliating.

Many of the industrial and agricultural chemicals, including certain fuels, petro-chemically derived plastics, PCBs (components of electrical installation), DDT, pesticides and growth hormones fed to animals, are actually oestrogen-like in their make-up. Called xenoestrogens (foreign oestrogens), they are in the foods we eat, the water we drink, even the air we breathe. Even though some of these chemicals are now banned, their residues are in the soil and, in the case of DDT for example, are still present in our bodies. PCBs permeate the planet and have been found in the fat cells of whales and seals in the arctic — virtually as far from civilisation as possible.

Being similar in their molecular structure to bodily oestrogen, the oestrogen receptor sites have difficulty differentiating between xeno-estrogens and natural oestrogens. Ill-matched as they may be, the receptor sites accept them and this fact links them to the worrying increase in reproductive disorders in males and females.

FERTILITY IS DROPPING

World-wide, fertility levels are dropping alarmingly and reproductive disorders such as endometriosis, PMS, breast cancer, and prostate cancer are on the increase. Increased infertility is now clearly linked to environmental pollutants. Danish, French, and Scottish studies have all shown sharp declines in sperm quality among European men in recent years.[11] Researchers have concluded that the decline in male reproductive health is caused by the exposure of the foetus to oestrogen-mimicking pollutants. Among the more common oestrogenic pollutants involved are DDT, aldrin, dieldrin, PCBs, dioxins, and furans.

Diethylstilbestrol (DES), a synthetic oestrogen which was prescribed to some five million pregnant women (to prevent miscarriage) between the late 1940s and the late 1970s, has also been found to cause abnormalities in the reproductive organs of males whose mothers took the drug. The researchers warn that it may take 20 to 40 years before a mother's exposure to oestrogenic pollutants manifests itself in her son in the form of poor sperm quality or abnormalities of the reproductive organs.[12]

We can reduce our exposure to oestrogen-mimicking chemicals by:
- Eating only organic foods.
- Avoiding the use of plastics in our homes (xeno-oestrogens

leach into food heated or stored in plastic).
- Avoiding taking synthetic oestrogens (HRT and the pill).
- Avoiding inhaling aromatic hydrocarbons from petrol or car exhaust.

Whatever the cause, too much oestrogen can mean not enough progesterone, and lack of ovulation means no progesterone. There is growing evidence and experience that adding progesterone in a form that is identical to that produced by the ovaries can in many cases reverse the disorders listed above.

PROPERTIES OF PROGESTERONE

Progesterone is what is known as a precursor hormone. Oestrogen is not. Progesterone is converted by the body into many other hormones as required, such as androstenedione, testosterone, and oestrogen. Progesterone is produced by the ovaries. It is also made by the adrenal glands in men and women and by the testes in men.

Progesterone is most commonly prescribed as a cream but is also available as an oil and in lozenge or micronised oral form. The cream is rubbed on to the soft tissue areas of the body. It bypasses the liver when applied to the skin and appears to be absorbed effectively this way. It is most readily and easily absorbed by the thinner-skinned areas of the body where there are plenty of capillaries. These include places where we tend to blush. The best areas therefore are the face, neck, and chest, along with the abdomen and upper and inner areas of arms and thighs. It is best to rotate the sites, applying the cream to one area one day and another the next. The recommended daily amount is 20mg. Available creams offer differing amounts. A 50-gram pot of cream that has 1 gram of progesterone in a vanishing base will provide the recommended 20mg in a quarter of a teaspoon.

Progesterone is stored in the fat cells and also adheres to the cell wall, so is not always locatable in a blood (serum level) test. However, with continued use, fat levels of progesterone reach an equilibrium and then levels increase in the blood, often resulting in more noticeable effects and benefit. For this reason, it may take two or three months of applying progesterone before you experience maximum benefit.

It is recommended that you apply progesterone cream in such a way that it mimics the monthly cycle. That is, if you are still menstruating, do not use it in the first half of the month when oestrogen is the predominant hormone. Wait until day 12 of your cycle to begin use and then stop when menstruation begins. If you are no longer menstruating, that is, you are post-menopausal or you have had a hysterectomy, then use the cream for three consecutive weeks each month.

NATURAL PROGESTERONE AND WILD YAM ARE NOT THE SAME THING

Natural progesterone is derived from the wild yam. The wild yam is a plant that is high in a plant hormone called diosgenin, which is similar in molecular structure to the progesterone produced by the ovaries. Although wild yam can have beneficial effects if taken as a supplement or applied as a cream, there is no evidence that the body can convert the plant hormone diosgenin to the human hormone progesterone.

Pharmaceutical companies have for years cultivated the wild yam, isolated the hormonal compounds, and used them as a base product to then convert them to synthetic versions of oestrogen and progesterone for use in the oral contraceptive pill and in hormone replacement therapy. These are patentable products because they are not identical to what occurs in nature. (Natural products, on the other hand, cannot be patented, so pharmaceutical companies generally show little interest in funding research programmes. This is a plausible explanation for the lack of research into natural progesterone, particularly since 1960 when synthetic progesterone became available. The focus then diverted to the progestins and progestagens produced in the laboratory.)

The 'natural' progesterone we are discussing here is natural in that it is identical in its molecular structure to what the ovaries produce in the second half of the monthly cycle, but it is created from disogenin in a laboratory. It is important to understand this because (a) it makes clear the difference between wild yam cream and natural progesterone cream; and (b) it is then understood that it is a *form* of hormone replacement — even if it is 'natural'.

SIDE-EFFECTS

Natural progesterone appears to be very safe. However, it is always wise to go by the stated dose. In excessive amounts it can make you sleepy. There is new evidence that in some women it can build up to abnormally high levels and with continued use be linked to weight gain and mild to moderate depression.[13] These women would show high levels of progesterone in saliva testing. It may be better in this instance to take it in an oral form, which doesn't have this effect. Dr Tessa Jones of Wellington, who has used natural progesterone in her practice for some years with good success, cautions her patients about this but admits that she has never witnessed such side-effects.

Because progesterone is a 'precursor' hormone, that is, it can be converted into other hormones, and because it is natural to the body, it is postulated that the body in most cases will either use it in this way or pass it out via the liver if more is applied than is required.

A small percentage of women may apparently notice signs of 'oestrogen dominance' when the cream is first applied. This may initially heighten the symptoms such as mood changes, fluid retention and breast tenderness. This normally subsides over two or three weeks.

WHERE CAN YOU GET THE CREAM?

Until recently, natural progesterone cream was available over the counter in certain health-food stores or through multi-level market distributors who were selling creams imported from the USA. Recent restrictions applied by the Ministry of Health has meant that the creams are now only officially available in New Zealand on prescription. If your doctor is uncertain where to order the cream, several compounding pharmacists are now making it available in the major cities (see Resources, page 224). Personal supplies can still be ordered via the internet, but product quality can vary. Check that you are getting a good product by reading the recommended list in John Lee's book *What Your Doctor May Not Tell You About Menopause*.

The following story demonstrates how effective natural progesterone can be for some women. At the age of 47, Ruth suddenly experienced some distressing symptoms of menopause. She felt a severe 'dizzy' or light-headed sensation a lot of the time, gained 6 kg in a month, and had aching legs and feet to the extent that it was sometimes difficult to walk or sleep.

'My breast size increased from a C cup to DD, my skin became dull and papery, and I had more migraine headaches than usual. These were acute, lasting for one to two days and causing four to six hours of vomiting. Over the next three months things continued to get worse. I had two full weeks of strong PMS (fluid retention and sore breasts, feeling tense and emotional), with the addition of some 'spotting' at day 17 of my cycle. I felt really unwell in the days before my period came, my face appearing to turn white or even green!

I was starting to feel depressed and unable to cope with everyday tasks and I was finally very shocked when my full period arrived at day 17. I waited until it finished then went to my doctor for help. He arranged for a lot of tests, made an appointment with a gynaecologist, and put me on a high dose of evening primrose oil.

'I attended a menopause seminar and read two of the suggested books, after which I changed my diet to include more fresh and plant-hormone-rich food. As soon as I reached day 12 in my cycle I started using natural progesterone cream.

'I noticed a slight but definite improvement with the evening

primrose oil and dietary changes, but immediately felt better when I applied the natural progesterone. I still felt odd, but better; and my skin quickly returned to normal.

'The next month my cycle was only 13 days and my periods had become heavier so from then I used the cream from day 5–25 each month. I started to notice a definite change for the better. I eventually gave up the evening primrose and some of the dietary changes but things continued to improve. The gynaecologist said my blood tests were "superb" and I am a health-conscious vegetarian, so my problem was probably just hormone imbalance. After two months on the progesterone cream I felt well enough to really enjoy my exercise again, and with no attempt to watch calories I lost 4 kg, and have lost another kilogram since (though I am still overweight). The third month my breast size returned to normal, and now by the fourth month I no longer have any spotting and my periods are back to my normal two days and occurring every 25 days. I have very little PMS now and continue to feel better and better. My headaches are fewer and I sleep very well.

'In retrospect I have probably suffered from oestrogen dominance all my life — we grew up in the country in the days of DDT etc, and I menstruated at 11 and my sister at 9 years old. I have had migraines and a monthly week of PMS since then until recent years. But now, after things suddenly started to get really bad, I feel back in control of my health and hopeful of continued well-being. For me it has been as good as magic!'

Jill's gynaecological history reads like a horror story. She is one of those women whose body cannot tolerate oestrogen replacement, yet she responds remarkably well to natural progesterone. It took many years and her own investigation to uncover this fact. After suffering for years with fibroids and endometriosis, Jill was given a hysterectomy at the age of 36, and an ovary was removed at the same time. Depression set in almost immediately along with pelvic pain, severe night sweats and hot flushes. She was given oestrogen replacement and proceeded to gain 17 kilos in three months. Her hair started falling out and she had continual ear and sinus infections. After two years her second ovary was removed and a different oestrogen dose prescribed. She then developed bowel pain, lost more hair, her blood pressure increased, and she had terrible back and neck pain, intense headaches, fluid retention, low libido and depression. Her weight stabilised at 19 kilos more than normal. Her doctor tried to help by adjusting the HRT dose — to no avail.

> 'I did a search on the internet and as I started reading about hormone imbalance I realised that everything I had suffered in my past right back to puberty was connected! I began to use natural progesterone along with the oestrogen — with the guidance of my doctor who felt I would still need oestrogen. There was quite an improvement but the symptoms, which I now realised to be oestrogen dominance, remained. I changed to a natural oestrogen cream (rather than synthetic) but it didn't help either.
>
> 'Finally I threw the oestrogen away totally, continued with progesterone only, and didn't look back. Within two months my hair grew back, the fluid retention went, blood pressure was normalised, I lost 5 kg, my headaches stopped, so did my sore back and neck, and I began to feel so much happier and healthier. My skin improved and the bowel pain was gone!
>
> 'Now, nine months later, even though I have had a few minor setbacks, I am still 100 times better than I was before I began using natural progesterone.'

OTHER HORMONES: DHEA, TESTOSTERONE, OESTROGEN AND MELATONIN

After menopause, it is not just oestrogen and progesterone levels that drop; another type of hormones called androgens also decreases in production by as much as 50 per cent. The main androgen hormones are testosterone, dehydroepiandrosterone

(DHEA) and androstenedione. DHEA is one of the body's most significant hormones and is the most abundant hormone in a young adult. But levels decline rapidly with age. Women with high levels of DHEA are known to have less breast cancer and osteoporosis.[14] DHEA is produced by the adrenal glands, which are located on top of the kidneys.

Testosterone is a predominantly male hormone, but it is present in women in small amounts and has important effects. It is produced by the ovaries and the adrenal glands. Like other hormones it declines with advancing years. It increases energy and libido and may offer protection against heart disease. It also has a bone-building capacity in both men and women.[15]

Current research suggests that supplemental DHEA may be valuable in preventing and treating cardiovascular disease, diabetes, obesity, cancer, immune system disorders and chronic fatigue.[16, 17] It is also currently being investigated as an anti-ageing hormone. Like progesterone, initial research indicates that DHEA may be helpful in treating osteoporosis. Application of DHEA as a cream by a group of 14 women over a one-year period showed an average increase in bone density of 2 per cent. The women also noticed an improvement in menopause-related signs, plus an improvement in well-being.[18] DHEA is now available (on prescription) as a cream in a nature-identical form. Topical testosterone is similarly available in a nature-identical cream form and may be helpful in treating low libido or sex drive.[19]

There may be other ways to increase flagging hormone levels. The revitalising effects of meditation and relaxation have already been noted. A study measured the DHEA levels in the blood of 423 people who practised Transcendental Meditation (TM) and compared them with 1253 people who did not. The ages ranged from 20 to 81 years. The effects of diet, obesity and exercise were statistically ruled out. Depending on the age range, the TM practitioners had levels of DHEA that were as high as members of the control group who were five to ten years younger.[20] It is believed that reduced hormone secretions may be due to free-radical cell damage. It follows, therefore, that if stress causes free radicals, and free radicals reduce the level of hormones, then meditation, which reduces stress, will assist in reversing the process.

NATURAL OESTROGEN REPLACEMENT

Oestrogen replacement in a nature-identical form is similarly available on prescription as a cream. It is usually offered in a dosage that replicates the oestrogens produced by the ovaries, that is, oestriol 2.0mg, oestradiol 0.25mg and oestrone 0.25mg on a daily basis. Some doctors prefer not to include oestrone, which is the more potent of the three.

MELATONIN

Melatonin is a regulatory hormone produced by a pea-sized region deep within the brain known as the pineal gland. Our bodies manufacture melatonin from seratonin, which is found in highest concentration in the pineal gland. Melatonin is produced while we sleep. Direct sunlight suppresses melatonin secretion, and interrupting sleep with very bright light can shut off its production. Travelling across time zones can cause the complaint known as jet lag, as the timing mechanism that triggers the pineal gland to produce melatonin is disrupted.

Melatonin production decreases as we age. It has been prescribed to treat stress, diabetes, heart disease, osteoporosis, immune function, headaches, jet lag, SAD (seasonal affective disorder), poor digestion, etc.[21, 22] There is increasing evidence that it may be useful in the treatment of breast cancer[23] and it has been shown to have potent anti oxidant capability.[24] Increasing interest in the role of melatonin and its application in the ageing population has led medical practitioners to begin prescribing it. It is available in New Zealand on prescription only, is banned in Canada, and can be purchased over the counter in the USA.

SUMMARY

'Nature-identical' hormone replacement or therapy is relatively new and we don't know the effects of long-term use. Many more studies are underway as interest in faithful replacement of physiologic hormone levels grows. It offers many women an attractive alternative to HRT. But it is still hormone therapy, and some women may prefer to approach mid-life health issues from a nutritional and lifestyle point of view. It is a decision largely affected by personal circumstance and preference.

7
OSTEOPOROSIS

The facts are worrying. New advances in technology to measure bone density reveal that New Zealand, along with the US and Sweden, has the highest rate of osteoporosis in the world. Seemingly a disease of the modern Western world, osteoporosis now afflicts about 25 per cent of elderly women in New Zealand. The current mid-life generation is shaping up to have the highest rate of the disease ever recorded. From the age of 50, women have a 40 per cent chance of having a fracture associated with osteoporosis. It is mystifying that the incidence of the disease has become so much worse in recent years.

Osteoporosis is an extremely painful disorder, which can bring with it disability and early death. The average life expectancy after a fracture from the age of 75 years is only six months. Men are not immune either. Around 12 per cent of men over 50 years have similar fractures. Although heart disease is the biggest killer of women after the age of 75 years, more women die from osteoporosis than they do of breast cancer, cervical cancer and uterine cancer put together.

IT IS TREATABLE!

If you find yourself at risk for osteoporosis, don't be discouraged. By eliminating risk factors you can prevent further deterioration, and there are many practical steps you can take to rebuild bone strength. New encouraging research shows that correct diet, mineral supplementation, hormone treatment, and regular exercise can reverse the trend of bone loss.

WHAT IS OSTEOPOROSIS?

Osteoporosis occurs when the bone becomes weakened and easily fractured. The bones of the vertebral column may be unable to support the weight of the body and may partially collapse — resulting in height reduction, stooping, and often intense pain due to pressure on the nerves entering and leaving the spinal column. Other bones easily fractured during falls are those of the wrist, hip and the neck of the femur (the long bone of the upper leg).

Our bones can seem to be like our teeth — passive and unchanging — but they are in fact living tissue richly supplied with blood vessels, nerve fibres and bone cells. Bone is constantly rebuilding while old bone is reabsorbed by the body. The adult skeleton is replaced entirely every seven to ten years.

Bone is made up of a framework or 'matrix' of interlocking fibres of the protein collagen. Collagen is normally flexible and is important in the structure of skin and nails. In bone, however, it is made strong and rigid by tiny crystals of calcium being deposited on it. Osteoporosis develops as a result of loss of bone matrix and calcium.

Bones contain cells called osteoclasts, which break down old or damaged bone cells, while osteoblasts work to replace the damaged bone. Osteoporosis occurs when the osteoblasts cannot replace lost bone tissue as fast the osteoclasts break it down.

Bone loss is the result of many factors, not just a lack of calcium in the diet. Studies have shown that the bone matrix requires a range of nutrients to maintain its strength. The typical Western diet with its high proportion of refined sugar, white flour, processed food and fat contains far less vitamins and minerals than are required for healthy bones. Nutritional requirements may also be increased by genetic factors, or metabolic changes at menopause. Oestrogen and progesterone depletion has been shown to accelerate the rate of bone loss. Excess protein in the form of meat and dairy products can create an acidic condition in the blood, which then extracts neutralising calcium from the bones. The calcium is lost in the urine when protein waste is excreted.

THE RISK FACTORS FOR OSTEOPOROSIS ARE:

- Lack of exercise/immobility
- Genetic conditions
- Inadequate levels of hydrochloric acid in the stomach
- Intestinal malabsorption
- Calcium, magnesium and mineral deficiency
- Vitamin deficiency (D, K, C or B_6)
- Decreased hormone production
- Caffeine (which is acidic and binds with alkaline calcium)
- Corticosteroid drugs
- Fluoridated water
- Cigarette smoking
- Alcohol
- Stress
- Phosphates in carbonated drinks
- Eating disorders
- Excessive exercising
- Menstrual irregularity
- Excessive meat protein in the diet

THE CAUSE OF OSTEOPOROSIS

The actual cause of osteoporosis is insufficient calcium being deposited in the bone matrix. There are several reasons for this:

- Not enough calcium, magnesium and other minerals in food.
- Enough calcium in the diet, but poor absorption from the gut. Most people only absorb about 40–60 per cent of the calcium they eat, and some appear to absorb much less.
- Too much calcium being excreted in the urine.
- A nutritionally deficient diet.

Calcium absorption can vary greatly. In healthy women, levels of absorption of calcium taken into the body can vary from 10 per cent to 70 per cent, so that even if the diet appears to be adequate in calcium, it may not ever reach the bone where it is most needed.

There are many factors that can trigger bone loss. Some drugs like oral corticosteroids such as cortisone and prednisone taken for illnesses such as asthma and rheumatoid arthritis can lead to substantial bone loss.[1] However, it has been found that supplementing with 1000mg of elemental calcium per day and 500 IU of vitamin D will prevent this loss.[2, 3]

Hormonal conditions such as an overactive thyroid or diabetes may affect bone density too. Research has shown that women taking higher doses of thyroid hormone are at risk for accelerated osteoporosis.[4] Oestrogen therapy (HRT) appears to prevent the bone loss associated with thyroid hormone use.

Smoking is known to be a factor. Research conducted in Melbourne found that women who smoke half a pack of cigarettes a day will, by the time of menopause, have a 5–10 per cent lower bone density than non-smokers. It is estimated that a 10 per cent decrease in bone density corresponds to a 44 per cent increase in the risk of hip fracture.[5]

Heavy drinking of alcohol increases body acidity, which in turn leaches calcium. Carbonated drinks high in phosphoric acid restrict calcium absorption. Researchers at Harvard Medical School have found that cola drinks increase the fracture rate in young girls in the US.[6]

When excessive exercise or eating disorders affect the menstrual cycle and periods stop, the subsequent lower levels of oestrogen and progesterone will in turn reduce bone density. These women are at greater risk of developing osteoporosis than women of average weight.

Research conducted at the University of Auckland has found that people carrying more weight have stronger and denser bones than thin people and are therefore less likely to suffer fractures and osteoporosis. The researchers found that the link between fat and bone density was because of higher levels of the hormones insulin and amylin circulating in fatter people. A similar protein hormone, adrenomedullin — produced by the adrenal glands — also helps increase bone density.[7]

Interestingly, countries with the highest consumption of meat protein and dairy products have the highest incidence of hip fractures and osteoporosis. Osteoporosis is most common in Caucasian women, less common in Asians, and least common in black women.[8] Statistics show that following a hip fracture, 50 per cent of women will not walk on their own again and 25 per cent will die within one year.[9] The reason for this is resulting medical complications and the effects of immobility on mental and physical health.

It is known that fluoride supplementation may increase bone mineral density, but it is also known that it increases fracture risk. Fluoridated water may therefore be a factor in increased incidence of hip fractures. In a recent medical letter, Dr John Lee MD says the following: 'Fluoride is toxic to collagen production, affecting not only the quantity but the quality of the collagen. In the presence of fluoride, the microarchitecture of collagen fibres is disordered, leading to a lack of tensile strength. After thirty years of studying the effects of fluoride on humans, I believe that this is the main cause of the increased incidence of hip fractures in communities with fluoridated water.'[10]

Our bone density continues to increase up to the age of 30. From then on it begins to decrease gradually for males and females until women reach their menopausal years when bone density drops rapidly by a dramatic 15 per cent. (Men continue to lose it gradually, hence the lesser risk.) Most at risk for osteoporosis are those who have low bone density before menopause. It is probably a good idea to take advantage of the new readily available low-radiation technology DEXA (dual energy X-ray absorptiometry) which will determine bone mineral density, and whether you are currently at risk. The risk of fractures increases with time and for most people the high-risk years are from the age of 75 years, so mid-life is the time to take serious steps to prevent it.

WHAT YOU CAN DO

One of the most important things to do to prevent osteoporosis is to start a walking or exercise programme. It is one thing to put calcium into our bodies, but actually getting it into our bones is another. Exercise — particularly weight bearing — forces the bones to take up available calcium. Therefore, calcium supplementation and exercise must go together.

Our bones, particularly in the spine and legs, are constantly remodelling and strengthening themselves as a result of stresses put on them by activity and gravity. Research shows that the pull of the muscles on the bones during weight-bearing exercise stimulates the bone-building cells (osteoblasts) to become more active and thereby increase bone density. Inactivity can be disastrous. Simple bed rest during recovery from illness can cause rapid resorption of bone to the point that fractures sometimes occur just lifting people from bed. Astronauts quickly lose bone density in a weightless environment.

Our lifestyle has changed enormously — technology is designed to take the weight off us, literally. We drive rather than walk, have power steering in our cars, throw our clothes in the dryer, turn on the dishwasher, switch on the oven (no more carting coal!) and chop and grate in the food processor. Work often involves long hours at a computer screen, and evening entertainment is beamed to us as we curl up in our living rooms.

Most of us are aware of the need for exercise, but without it naturally occurring in day-to-day activities, we have to make a conscious effort to attend the gym, ride a bike, walk to the store and carry home the groceries. It is vital, therefore, to take reasonably intense exercise at least three times a week. Brisk walking is one of the best forms of exercise, as is dancing, cycling, jogging, and playing tennis.

CALCIUM

Calcium is an essential nutrient for normal growth and development and most adults need to consume 1200–2000mg per day. Today's average for most women is only 500mg. By eating wild plants, our Stone Age ancestors ate from 2000–3000mg of calcium per day. It is not surprising that our bones are becoming so fragile.

Ninety-nine per cent of the total body calcium is found in the bones and teeth. The one per cent circulating in the blood has significant functions, however. Calcium helps regulate heartbeat, nervous system function, muscle control, enzyme systems, and hormone secretions, and helps cells to cohere and blood to coagulate. If the body does not have enough circulating calcium for these functions, it leaches it from the bones, eventually leading to osteoporosis. Research has also shown that excess free radicals are involved in leaching of bone calcium. Keeping your dietary antioxidant intake high, and your stress levels low can help to protect the body's bone structure.[11]

DIETARY SOURCES OF CALCIUM AND OTHER ESSENTIAL MINERALS

It is best to try and get as much calcium as you can from your diet. The best natural sources of calcium are the alkaline mineral-rich foods like fruits, green leafy vegetables, and sea vegetables or seaweeds. Seaweeds contain high amounts of calcium, phosphorus, magnesium, boron, iron, iodine and sodium. They also contain vitamins A, B_1, C and E, and are one of the few vegetarian sources of vitamin B_{12}. There are some delicious seaweeds available in New Zealand now. You can add them to soups, stir fries, stews and pizzas or eat them with sushi or other rice dishes (see Recipes, page 192).

Milk and dairy products are high in calcium but are not necessarily helpful, despite repeated assurances from the dairy industry. We are after all the generation who grew up suffering the daily ordeal of half a pint of warm milk at school. It has not made us less at risk for osteoporosis! The latest research indicates that in the daily diet the ratio of calcium to magnesium should be about 2:1. In milk, the ration of calcium to magnesium is 8:1, which may prevent effective absorption of calcium into bone.[12]

Foods that are high in calcium are:
- Leafy green vegetables — particularly bitter salad vegetables like rocket and mesclun
- Chinese leafy greens like pak choy, broccoli, parsley, spinach and silver beet
- Sea vegetables — wakame, karengo, nori, kelp (kombu), hijiki and arame
- Tofu and soy milk
- Pulses and legumes — black peas, chickpeas, pinto beans, lentils
- Dairy products — non-fat yoghurt, trim milk, fresh cheeses like feta and cottage cheese
- Canned sardines or salmon (with bones)
- Nuts — almonds, Brazil nuts, hazelnuts
- Sesame seeds

PHYTOESTROGENS
Initial studies into the effects of phytoestrogens like soy isoflavones on bone density suggest that they have oestrogen-like activity with regard to bone metabolism and may produce a significant increase in bone mineral density when included in the diet.[13]

WHICH CALCIUM SUPPLEMENT IS BEST?
Some forms of calcium are more easily absorbed than others. Calcium citrate and calcium maleate are much better absorbed

than calcium carbonate, which requires very good levels of stomach acid. Calcium absorption can be improved by taking calcium supplements in divided doses with meals, or last thing at night. People with a tendency to form kidney stones should preferably use calcium citrate as a supplement.[14] Calcium hydroxyapatite is an excellent source of the nutrients needed for bone formation. However, vegetarians need to be aware that it is derived from beef or calf bone. In addition, in the days of animal-borne diseases it could involve that risk.

A New Zealand study conducted at Auckland University in 1993 confirmed that calcium supplementation reduced bone density loss by 43 per cent. In an editorial accompanying the study it was recommended that women increase their daily calcium intake to 1500mg combined with a daily intake of 400–800 IU of vitamin D.[15]

A 1998 placebo-controlled, double-blind study involving 389 men and women over 65 years of age evaluated the effect of supplementation with calcium and vitamin D. Half the group took 500mg of calcium citrate maleate and 700 IU (17.5 micrograms) of vitamin D daily at bedtime while the other half took placebos. At the end of the three-year study period participants who had taken calcium and vitamin D supplements had increased their bone mineral density significantly and also reported far fewer fractures.[16]

There is evidence that dietary calcium may lower blood pressure and cholesterol levels (in men), help prevent the development of diabetes, and protect against colon and rectal cancer.

MAGNESIUM AND CALCIUM MUST GO TOGETHER

As much as 50 per cent of all the magnesium in the body is found in the bones. Many researchers are now reporting that magnesium deficiency plays a big part in the development of osteoporosis. Studies have shown that women suffering from osteoporosis tend to have a lower intake of magnesium than normal and also have lower levels of magnesium in their bones. A magnesium deficiency can also affect the production of the biologically active form of vitamin D and thereby further promote osteoporosis. A trial in Israel showed that postmenopausal women with osteoporosis could stop further bone loss by supplementing with 250–750mg/day of magnesium for two years.[17] Some (8 per cent) even experienced a significant increase in bone density. Another experiment in Czechoslovakia found that 65 per cent of women who supplemented with 1500–3000mg of magnesium lactate daily for two years completely got rid of their pain and stopped further development of deformities of the vertebrae.[18]

You need at least half as much magnesium as you do calcium. The optimum intake of magnesium is 600–1000mg and of calcium is 1200–2000mg. Your body needs an adequate supply of all the minerals found in bone, which is virtually all the minerals found in food. The absence of any one of these could stop the bone regeneration process.

MINERALS...

- Manganese — a trace mineral, which is required for bone mineralisation and the formation of connective tissue in cartilage and bone. Hair analysis has revealed significantly lower levels of manganese in subjects with osteoporosis.[19]

- Zinc, along with vitamin A and C, is essential for the formation of collagen. It enhances the biochemical action of vitamin D. Zinc levels have been found to be low in elderly people with osteoporosis. Zinc is found in wholegrain products, wheat bran and germ, brewer's yeast and pumpkin seeds.

- Boron improves the metabolism of calcium and magnesium and also increases the level of oestrogens in some women. In a 1987 study, women taking 3mg of supplemental boron for seven weeks lost 44 per cent less calcium and 33 per cent less magnesium in their urine than those women in the study not taking boron.[20] Boron is found in alfalfa and seaweeds.

- Silicon — important in the formation of connective tissue, bone and cartilage. It combines with calcium in osteoblasts and is highly concentrated at sites of growing bones. It is found in hard unprocessed grains and vegetables. Horsetail tea and oatstraw are excellent sources of silica. It is beneficial to drink one cup per day.

- Strontium (the trace mineral — not to be confused with the radioactive substance of the same name) plays a crucial role in bone remodelling. It tends to migrate to sites in bone where active remodelling is taking place.

- Copper is a cofactor in the strengthening of connective bone tissue.

AND VITAMINS ETC...

- Vitamin D. The best source is sunlight on the skin. Vitamin D intake is important as it enhances calcium absorption. The body converts vitamin D to its biologically active form vitamin D_3. This process requires magnesium. A study conducted in Dunedin in 1992 measuring 400 postmenopausal women over a three-year period found that spinal fractures were three times lower in the group taking Vitamin D than in the group taking calcium alone.[21]

- Vitamins A and C are used by your body to make collagen, which keeps bones flexible and strong. Studies have shown that osteoporosis can result from vitamin C deficiency.

- Vitamin K is required for the production of osteocalcin, a protein that attracts calcium to bone tissue and facilitates beneficial calcium crystal formation.

- Pyroxidine (vitamin B_6) is required for collagen linking and the strength of connective bone tissue.

- Betain. Individuals with osteoporosis often absorb calcium poorly. Low stomach acid (hypochlorhydria) is relatively common in women over the age of 50 and may reduce absorption of most forms of calcium. Betain increases the absorption of bone-building nutrients.

Fortunately you can now buy calcium products that include most or all of these in one capsule. It is a good idea to take calcium supplements last thing at night before bed, as the body will absorb it most effectively during sleep. It is also calming and will help you to sleep.

EVENING PRIMROSE OIL (GLA)

Recent developments indicate that essential fatty acids (EFAs) may be important in rebuilding bone. EFAs have been shown to play an important role in a wide range of diseases including skin problems, arthritis, inflammation, heart and circulation disorders, some psychiatric disorders and premenstrual syndrome among others. Research has shown that GLA supplementation (in the form of evening primrose oil) increases calcium intake, reduces calcium excretion and puts calcium into a strengthened bone matrix.[22]

HORMONES AND OSTEOPOROSIS

Osteoporosis is also associated with the age-related decline of hormones that occurs in both men and women. These hormones, which include oestrogen, progesterone, DHEA, testosterone and human growth hormone, monitor the breakdown of old bone cells and the building up of new ones. When the two processes are in balance, bone density is stable, but when more bone is broken down than is built up — which is often what happens when hormone levels drop — osteoporosis occurs. Supplementing with these hormones has been found to slow down, and in some cases rebuild lost bone.

HORMONE REPLACEMENT THERAPY

Oestrogen signals osteoclasts (bone-eating cells) when to die. When oestrogen levels are low, as they are after menopause, osteoclasts live longer and continue to break down bone. Supplemental oestrogen has therefore been found to slow down bone density loss. The risk of hip fracture has been found to be reduced in women currently or recently using HRT. Current users can reduce their risk of hip fracture by about 70 per cent. Women using combined oestrogen and progestagen have less risk than those using oestrogen alone. However, within five years of stopping HRT the benefit ceases. [23, 24]

A new development in the application of HRT has been to start women nine or more years after the menopause, which gives reduction as good as starting it earlier. This lessens the years of constant use. Long-term use of HRT increases the risk of breast cancer, and the risk of endometrial cancer is not completely eliminated.

NATURAL PROGESTERONE

In initial research, natural progesterone has been shown to actually reverse the osteoporotic process and increase bone density. John R Lee, MD, followed 100 post-menopausal women with osteoporosis for a minimum of six years. They were treated with transdermal natural progesterone cream and a calcium, magnesium, boron, vitamin D, and vitamin C supplement. Some of the women were also taking oestrogen. Reduction in height stabilised in these women, bone pain disappeared, and no new fractures were noted. In the 63 patients who followed up with bone mineral density scans, their bone densities had increased by 15.4 per cent as opposed to the expected 4.5 per cent loss for that age group. Remarkably, this increase was as significant in women over 70 as in younger women. Progesterone stimulates osteoblasts, the cells that build new bone.[25, 26, 27] This was an observational study. A further clinical trial is underway at the Chelsea & Westminster Hospital in London.

Several New Zealand women have reported increases in bone mineral density since using natural progesterone cream. In two recent examples, an 83-year-old woman was found to have established osteoporosis in both hip and spine after a DEXA scan in 1997. After exactly one year of treatment with natural progesterone her bone density had increased significantly. And a 50-year-old woman whose spine showed degenerative change in the direction of osteoporosis was similarly found to show significant improvement after one year's use of natural progesterone.

DHEA

DHEA (dehydroepiandrosterone) is an important sex hormone secreted by the adrenal gland. It is converted into androgens and oestrogens in peripheral tissue. Its production peaks between the ages of 20–30 years and then declines rapidly with ageing. Application of DHEA as a cream by a group of 14 women over a one-year period showed an average increase in bone density of 2 per cent. The women also noticed an improvement in menopause-related signs plus an improvement in well-being.[28]

BISPHOSPHONATES

Drugs such as the bisphosphonates Fosomax, Alendronate, and Didronel inhibit the resorption of old bone and lead to an increase in bone mineral density. They are expensive, can have unpleasant side-effects, and are poorly absorbed by the gut. They may not be suitable for many women, and further development of these drugs is underway.

BONE MINERAL DENSITY TESTING

Bone density testing is a relatively new tool in the diagnosis of osteoporosis. Because you cannot accurately tell the state of people's bones by looking at them or even applying the known risk factors, testing is very helpful. Bone mineral density (BMD) varies depending on the size of a woman's bones and on the concentration of minerals in her bone. Despite the advances in measuring BMD, it has not been found to be a good predictor of fracture rate, which is after all what the concern is all about. That means that you may have low BMD, but never fracture, because your BMD is normal for you. If you have low BMD and have had previous fractures, however, you can be fairly certain that you are in the high-risk category. Other factors are important too in the elderly population, like balance, vision, muscle strength and coordination.

Bone density testing has revolutionised the diagnosis of osteoporosis but it doesn't bring all the answers and it does have limitations. The most common techniques are dual-energy X-ray absorptiometry (DEXA) and dual photon absorptiometry (DPA). An X-ray or photon (light) beam is directed at a site such as the hip or lumbar spine and the energy of the beam is measured as it exits from the body. The denser the bone, the greater the loss of beam energy. DEXA precision drops off as bone density becomes less, particularly in the elderly, in which case ultrasound may bring a better result.

OTHER TESTING TECHNIQUES

Calcium levels in urine can be tested to determine how much is being excreted in relation to absorption. A new test has recently been developed which will also measure the biochemicals excreted in the urine when bone breaks down. Both these tests can help to narrow the cause of low bone density.

Other than iron levels, blood tests cannot reveal mineral levels in the body. There is a simple alternative however. Hair mineral analysis tests a sample of your hair and analyses it for levels of calcium, magnesium, zinc, selenium, manganese, chromium and nickel, and identifies any deficiencies. It also provides valuable information about levels of toxic heavy metals such as arsenic, mercury, aluminium, lead and cadmium. This is an invaluable test as you can clearly see what supplementation is required to keep your bones strong, and action can be taken to reduce levels of heavy metals (see Resources, page 224).

8
BREAST CANCER

Breast cancer is an epidemic in our society. Four decades ago the breast cancer rate was one woman in 20. Now it is one in nine. It is the most common cause of death among women aged 40–50, and is increasing every year. Fifteen hundred New Zealand women are diagnosed with breast cancer every year, and six hundred of those women die of the disease.

Although the definitive answer to the cause of breast cancer continues to elude modern science, growing evidence reveals many risk factors, and many preventative measures. It is clear (as with most modern diseases) that major influencing factors are dietary and environmental. The following is a summary of the evidence that we have to date regarding the risk factors, and the known steps you can take to prevent getting breast cancer.

Risk factors for breast cancer:

- *Age*
  Breast cancer incidence increases with age. Eighty-five per cent

of breast cancers occur after the age of 45, and 67 per cent occur after the age of 50.[1]

- **Race**
  Western women — i.e., New Zealanders, North Americans, and Europeans, are five times more likely to develop breast cancer than Asian women.[2]

- ***Early menarche, late menopause***
  Women who started menstruating early or have a later than average menopause have an increased risk of breast cancer.[3]

- **Genetic**
  Although other factors appear to be more important in the development of breast cancer than inherited genes, about 10 per cent of cancers do appear to be family related. Women with mothers or sisters diagnosed with breast cancer are therefore at a higher relative risk.[4] But interestingly, a recent study found that young women with a family history of breast cancer are less at risk of dying of the disease than women with no such family history. The researchers speculate that this may be due in part to the less aggressive nature of the type of tumours common in genetically predisposed women.[5]

- ***Age at first full-term pregnancy***
  Giving birth before the age of 30 is associated with a slight reduction in breast cancer risk. Having no children also slightly increases the risk.[6]

- **Free radicals**
  Free-radical cell damage is caused by stress, environmental pollution in the form of pesticides and organochlorines, pharmaceuticals, processed foods, cigarette smoking, alcohol, and electromagnetic radiation — including excess exposure to sunlight. Antioxidants play a crucial role in controlling free-radical damage.

There is substantial evidence that free-radical attacks on DNA are a major factor in the development and spread (metastasis) of breast cancer. Researchers have found that women with metastasised breast cancer exhibit twice as much free-radical damage to the breast tissue as women with localised cancer.[7]

- *Polyunsaturated fat intake*
  In a very recent study, researchers in Sweden found that a high intake of polyunsaturated fats — particularly from margarine, breads and cereals — increased the risk of breast cancer by 69 per cent for every 5 g increment in daily intake.[8] Mono-unsaturated fats (olive oil in particular) have been found to be protective (see page 127).

- *Alcohol*
  Alcohol consumption is associated with an increase in breast cancer incidence, and even small amounts may increase the risk according to a recently published American study. In a meta-analysis of studies involving 322,647 women, researchers found that women who drank two to five alcoholic drinks a day had a 41 per cent increased chance of developing breast cancer compared to teetotallers. Even as little as one glass a day — whether beer, wine or other liquor — increased the risk by 9 per cent and the risk increased substantially with each subsequent drink. Avoiding alcohol consumption is therefore an obvious step in reducing breast cancer risk. The risk for cancer is also found to be increased in women who use alcohol and take oestrogen (HRT).[9]

- *Use of oral contraceptives*
  The main findings are that there is a small increase in the risk of having breast cancer diagnosed in current users of combined oral contraceptives and in women who had stopped use in the past 10 years, but there is no evidence of an increase in the risk more than 10 years after stopping use.[10]

- *Hormone replacement therapy*
  There is an increased risk of breast cancer for those women who have been using HRT for five or more years. Women who have used HRT for an average of 11 years have an increased risk of breast cancer of 35 per cent compared to women who have never used HRT. The increase in risk occurs in women who are currently using HRT or have used it within the last five years.[11] The risk becomes greater as you age. In a recent *Women's Health Update* Dr Charlotte Paul of Otago University summarised the results of the major report published in the *Lancet* in 1997: 'The absolute number of breast cancers developing between the ages of 50 and 70 among 1,000 women who have not used HRT, is about 45. The extra number of breast cancers occurring in women using HRT for five years from age 50 was estimated to be about two, for 10 years about six, and for 15 years' use about 12 cancers.'[12] Whether HRT affects the number of deaths from breast cancer is not known.

- *Being a flight attendant*
  Several studies have shown a doubling in the incidence of breast cancer amongst retired flight attendants in the US, Finland and Sweden. Suggested causes are radiation, or exposure to the organochlorine pesticide DDT, which was sprayed in aircraft from the 1950s to the 1970s.[13]

- *Smoking*
  Although not all studies have revealed a connection, a 1995 Danish study of 3240 women found that those who had smoked for 30 years or more had a 60 per cent increased risk of cancer compared with women who had never smoked. Smokers also tend to get breast cancer earlier.[14]

BREAST CANCER DETECTION

Despite its limitations, mammography is still the best tool for early detection of breast cancer, and has saved and extended the lives of thousands of women. Mammograms can detect breast cancers well before they can be felt, even smaller than one centimetre in size. They can detect close to 90 per cent of breast cancers. But they do miss 10–15 per cent of early breast cancers, thus providing a false sense of security in some cases.[15, 16] Of the 10 per cent undetected by mammography, most are obscured by dense breast tissue.

Mammography has been found to be most effective for women from the age of 50. Women in the younger age group from 40–49 years who have recognised risk factors for breast cancer may wish to consider regular screening too, although it is believed by many that there is little benefit generally in screening women under the age of 50, and that screening could have the potential to cause harm. A false positive result can cause great stress and lead to unnecessary biopsies and surgery. It is important to note also that hormone replacement therapy can increase the density of breast tissue, making mammography less reliable.[17] These women may need to include ultrasound in their screening programme. In New Zealand the national breast cancer screening programme BreastScreen Aotearoa now offers free mammograms every two years to women aged between 50 and 64.

Women under 50 are advised to self-examine their breasts and have their doctor examine their breasts once a year. A recent study showed that among women aged 40–49 there was a 56.2 per cent chance of having a false positive result after 10 mammograms. The study of 2400 women aged 40–69 showed that over a 10-year period, one-third of women who take part in mammography screening will need additional tests, even though breast cancer is not present, and the majority of the lesions or masses discovered will turn out to be benign.[18] To establish this fact the women involved have to go through additional diagnostic tests such as further mammography, ultrasound, fine needle aspiration or open surgical biopsy. These tests can be expensive and anxiety-provoking. Alternatives are being worked on. A team of researchers from eight European hospitals and universities reported very recently in the *Lancet* that a new electronic device called the Biofield Diagnostic System can provide accurate information as to whether an abnormal breast mass is cancerous or not.[19]

A blood test that will detect breast cancer is being developed but is unavailable at this time.

In an encouraging new development an American engineer has developed a temperature-sensitive pad that can be worn inside the bra for 15 minutes to record skin temperature across the breast. If an area of the breast shows a temperature 2°F higher or more than it does in the same area of the other breast, then there is probably a tumour present. Clinical trials have shown the device to be 80 per cent accurate in all women and 90 per cent accurate in women under 50 years. It is safer and more comfortable than mammography, but is not suitable for women who have had a mastectomy or lumpectomy or whose breasts are mismatched. More trials of the pads are underway. The cost is much less than mammography too.[20]

Early detection maximises the chances of a good recovery. It is important to seek medical advice if you notice any abnormal breast changes such as:

- Dimpling of the skin or any changes to breast texture or shape
- Changes to nipple shape or unexplained discharges
- Breast lumps or breast thickening
- Underarm tenderness or skin changes.

BREAST CANCER PREVENTION/TREATMENT

DIET IS VERY IMPORTANT FOR BREAST CANCER SURVIVAL

In recent years there has been evidence to link breast cancer with the type of foods we eat. Countries such as Japan where fat intake is low and the diet is composed of mainly vegetables, fish and rice have a low incidence of both breast cancer and benign breast disorders. Recent research from Australia reports that women with a high daily intake of phytoestrogens — particularly those found in soy products and whole grains, berries, flaxseed, fruit and vegetables — have a three- to four-fold lower risk of developing breast cancer than women with a low intake of these foods.[21, 22]

Japanese green tea has been found to reduce cancer risk in women too. Women who drink 10 or more cups a day have a 43 per cent lower risk of developing cancer. The researchers of this Japanese study conclude that the 'Strong potency of green tea . . . points us towards a new strategy of cancer chemoprevention without toxic effects'.[23]

Breast cancer is more prevalent in countries with a high overall fat intake, especially polyunsaturated fats. A very recent and massive Swedish study involving 61,000 women over six years found that a high intake of monounsaturated fat (for example, olive oil) is protective against breast cancer, while a high intake of polyunsaturated fats significantly increases the risk of breast cancer. The largest contributor to polyunsaturated fat intake was margarine. Interestingly, the researchers found no correlation between saturated fat intake (for example, butter) and breast cancer risk.[24]

A further study published in the *Journal of the National Cancer Institute* also found that olive oil reduces the risk of breast cancer. This study of Greek women found that in addition to the beneficial effects of olive oil, the women who ate the most fruit and vegetables had 48 per cent less breast cancer compared with the group who ate the least.[25]

Alpha-linolenic acid (also known as n-3 or Omega-3) is the essential fatty acid that is found in pumpkin seeds, flaxseeds, soybeans and walnuts, as well as oily fish such as wild salmon, mackerel, sardines and wild trout. A French study involving 121 women who had been diagnosed with localised breast cancer found that the cancer was more likely to spread to lymph nodes in women with a low level of alpha-linolenic acid in their tissue. The researchers concluded that dietary supplementation with alpha-linolenic acid may delay or prevent the development of metastases. The researchers also point out that a high dietary intake of fish oil helps prevent cancer and improves survival among breast cancer patients.[26]

ANTIOXIDANTS

A free radical is an oxygen molecule with a missing electron. Because it is extremely unstable as a result, it is highly reactive with other atoms and molecules, and can cause great damage. It can incapacitate nearly everything it touches including cell membranes and DNA.

Once again, nature offers a nutritional solution. Because they also have to defend themselves against free-radical damage, plants produce a rich source of antioxidant substances like vitamin C and E to control free radicals. Increasing your intake of fresh fruits and vegetables naturally increases your defences against free radicals as well as simultaneously providing you with phytoestrogens. Vitamin C is the most well known of the nutrient antioxidants, and it is probably a good idea to supplement daily. A study found that women who consumed more than 210 mg of vitamin C per day had a 57 per cent lower risk of dying from breast cancer than women who were getting less than 110 mg per day.[27] Remarkably, repeated clinical trials to measure the antioxidant properties of the ancient Ayur-Vedic formula of fruits and herbs called 'Amrit Kalash' have revealed it to be an antioxidant that is literally one thousand times more effective than vitamin E or vitamin C[28] (see Resources, page 224).

Other vitamins have been found to actually inhibit tumour growth — several fat-soluble vitamins, namely the vitamins A, D, E and K, have been found to be effective and to help increase survival if taken during chemotherapy and radiation therapy. Now researchers report that vitamin E succinate (d-alpha-tocopherol) actually kills aggressive types of breast cancer cells in vitro. They conclude that vitamin E supplementation may be of use in the treatment of aggressive human breast cancers.[29]

(Note: The 'd' designation in d-alpha-tocopherol indicates that it is a natural source of vitamin E derived from vegetable oil or wheatgerm. Natural vitamin E has been found to be far more effective than the form synthesised from a petroleum base.)

It has been found that a high dietary intake of vitamin A can reduce the risk of breast cancer by 50 per cent and that folic acid and fibre is important too.[30]

Beta-carotene is essential also. Women who have a relatively high intake of beta-carotene (up to 7690 IU per day) have been found to have half the risk of dying from breast cancer than women with a low intake (less than 3607 IU per day). More than 500 different carotenes have been identified — all with antioxidant properties. They are found in fruits and vegetables like red pepper, leafy dark green vegetables, pumpkin, and carrots.

Coenzyme Q10 or ubiquinol is a natural substance produced by the body. We tend to become deficient in it as we age. It is being hailed as one of the most important and effective antioxidants, with evidence that it may be effective in the fight against breast cancer. A Danish trial showed that tumours actually regressed and disappeared in patients supplementing with coenzyme Q10.[31] Coenzyme Q10 is found in seafood and organ meats. Supplements are easily absorbed by the body, especially if they are taken in combination with vegetable oil. The recommended daily dose is 30 mg, but higher doses are suggested for the treatment of diseases.

The trace mineral selenium, largely missing from New Zealand soil, is a powerful antioxidant and is an essential step in the body's production of glutathione peroxidase, an enzyme that neutralises free radicals. Studies in the US have shown that selenium supplementation helps prevent cancer and appears to inhibit the growth of tumours.[32, 33] Foods rich in selenium are grains (for example, wheat), sunflower seeds, and garlic that have been grown in selenium-rich soil. Seafood is a good source, and a very rich source is the Brazil nut — especially nuts straight from the shell.

LOWER EXPOSURE TO CHEMICAL POLLUTION

Although currently there are conflicting outcomes, some studies show a link between breast cancer and toxic organochlorines. These toxic chemicals abound in our environment — in the air, the soil and the water. They are among the most dangerous chemicals known to man and include PCBs, and the pesticides dioxin, DDE and DDT. They are oestrogen-like chemicals that interfere with naturally occurring oestrogen and have thus been suspected of a breast cancer link. They disperse easily into the environment and do not break down easily. A recent report from the Ministry for the Environment found that Auckland has higher levels of organochlorines than any other region of New Zealand.[34]

A recent analysis from the long-running Nurses Health Study in the USA does not support the theory that pesticides may cause cancer, and further research into environmental exposures has been called for. DDE (a DDT by-product) levels in women with breast cancer were actually found to be lower than those in the blood of matched controls, leading researchers to conclude that there was no association.[35] However, there have been many other studies that have drawn a link between organochlorines and cancer. An industrial accident in Germany exposed large numbers of women to the pesticide dioxin. These women are now experiencing a higher incidence of breast cancer, and twice the rate of cancer deaths as the whole German population.[36] When pesticides were banned in Israel in 1976, the breast cancer mortality rate, which had been steadily increasing before the ban, fell by 8 per cent in the decade following. There was a 34 per cent decrease in the incidence of breast cancer in women aged 25–34 over the 10-year period.[37]

The majority of pesticides we consume come from meat and vegetables. You can lower your exposure to these chemicals by eating organic food, decreasing your intake of meat and dairy foods, which store and concentrate these chemicals, and making sure your drinking water is uncontaminated. Taking antioxidant nutrients as well will protect you against further exposure and against the pesticides you already have stored in your body. A detoxifying and cleansing programme like Ayur-Vedic panchakarma or a detoxifying diet can be very helpful.

Do what you can to change the laws of the land which allow these levels of poisons to be in our environment. New Zealand currently tops the world list for breast cancer incidence, and at the same time we have appallingly high allowable levels of pesticide residue in our food and environment.

Just a warning — although we are currently free of it in New Zealand, beware the genetically engineered bovine growth hormone (rBGH or bST) which in the USA is injected into cows and subsequently makes its way into milk, yoghurt and other dairy products. It may well be marketed here and we could find ourselves subjected to yet another product that may raise our risk of cancer.

It is also extremely important to reduce your exposure to risk factors in the home environment. We now know that carcinogens abound in the form of household cleaners, cosmetics like talcum powder, hair dye and face make-up, garden weed killers and disinfectants. Read the whole story in Samuel Epstein and David Steinman's book, *The Breast Cancer Prevention Program*.[38]

THE ROLE OF HORMONES

Melatonin, a hormone secreted by the pituitary gland, has been shown to stop the growth of breast cancer tumours. An American laboratory study using human breast cancer cells found that when melatonin was administered in concentrations similar to those encountered during the night when melatonin production is at its peak, the tumour growth was inhibited.[39] A completely dark bedroom is required for optimum secretion of melatonin, and links are being made between electric light, electromagnetic exposure and lowered levels of natural melatonin. Dimmer lighting in the evenings is recommended prior to falling asleep.[40]

Melatonin is produced by the body, but it is known that St John's wort, feverfew, and the Chinese herb huang-qin (*Scutellaria biacalensis*) contain significant amounts of melatonin. Research has shown that consumption of herbs and edible plants containing melatonin increases the supply of circulating melatonin in mammals.[41]

More recent research reveals that the cancer-cell-killing effect of melatonin is dependent on the body producing adequate levels of the natural antioxidant glutathione.[42] Glutathione levels can be boosted by taking daily doses of 500 mg of vitamin C or taking the amino acid supplement glutamine. Selenium-rich foods such as Brazil nuts will stimulate glutathione production. Foods rich in glutathione are raw fruits and vegetables — namely avocado, watermelon, tomatoes, strawberries, grapefruit, boiled potatoes (with skin) and fresh cooked asparagus.

NATURAL PROGESTERONE

Progesterone also appears to have a protective role against breast cancer (see page 91).[43] At a recent world conference on the menopause, European specialists advocated the use of progestins that are as close as possible to natural progesterone in the treatment of breast cancer. They predicted that this was a treatment we would hear much more of in the future.[44]

Research is underway in Germany to find an appropriate type of progesterone to use in reducing breast cancer risk as preliminary studies show that natural progesterone will reduce breast cancer cell proliferation.[45]

GET SOME SUN

Sunlight in moderation is good for you and may actually prevent cancer rather than cause it. It is thought that the cancer-protecting effect of sunlight is related to its ability to produce vitamin D in the body.

TIMING IS CRITICAL IN BREAST CANCER SURGERY

A British study has shown that timing of breast cancer surgery in relation to the menstrual cycle is critical. Women who have surgery during the latter part of their menstrual cycle have a significantly better survival rate than do women who undergo surgery early in the cycle. Researchers at Guy's Hospital have found that when blood serum levels of progesterone are highest — that is, during the second half of the cycle, a woman has a 76 per cent better survival rate. Operating when progesterone levels are highest is also important in cases where lymph nodes are involved in the cancer. Here the survival rate was twice as good.[46]

EXERCISE AND BREAST CANCER

Yet another good reason to keep exercising. Recent studies of Norwegian and Finnish women showed that women who exercised regularly had less risk of breast cancer. The risk reduction was greater in younger women than older women, and the risk was lowest for leaner women who exercised at least four times a week, and for women who had higher levels of physical activity at work.[47]

MIND–BODY MEDICINE

The mind–body relationship is becoming more accepted by the medical establishment along with the positive effects of relaxation therapy and visualisation on the immune system. It has been found that relaxing and imagining a powerful immune system can actually increase T-cell levels. Researchers reported that women with metastatic breast cancer who participated in group therapy as part of their treatment survived twice as long as women who received medical treatment but no group therapy.[48]

STRESS MANAGEMENT

The mind and body are interrelated. Thoughts create physical responses. If we feel anxious about something, for example, our body responds and gives us 'butterflies' in the stomach as a result of the biochemicals that our thinking creates. Stress is one of the major factors in the creation of free radicals — the unstable molecules that cause physical damage to cells. Excessive free radicals are known to cause cancer and other diseases. Studies have shown that breast cancer spreads more quickly among women who have repressed personalities, feel hopeless and are unable to express anger, fear, and other negative emotions.[49]

As part of our own health maintenance and disease prevention it is essential that we practise some form of relaxation or meditation that will reduce stress, anxiety and tension. The most well researched of these is Transcendental Meditation or TM, known to be twice as effective as all other types of meditation and relaxation in relieving anxiety.[50] It is a purely mental technique, but by creating a relaxed and positive state of mind, it breaks the 'stress syndrome' and generates a corresponding different pattern of biochemicals in the body. A large health insurance study measuring 2000 practitioners of TM over a five-year period found that compared to a matched group, the TM meditators were hospitalised 55 per cent less for cancer and 87 per cent less for heart disease.[51]

OVARIAN CANCER AND TALCUM POWDER

One in every one hundred women will develop ovarian cancer in their lifetime. It is a form of cancer that can go undetected because of the difficulties associated with diagnosis. Now researchers at Yale University School of Medicine report that women who use talcum powder have a 42 per cent higher risk of developing ovarian cancer than non-users. The development of ovarian cancer is particularly likely if the talc is applied to the perineal area (the area between the anus and the vagina). One study has shown that about 75 per cent of all tumours actually contain talc particles.[52]

SUMMARY

The best way to dispel fear of breast cancer is through education and self-responsibility. Understanding the risk factors and the often-simple preventative steps available to you, like diet, exercise, and stress management allows you to take a proactive role in maintaining your good health.

9
WOMEN AND HEART DISEASE

We tend to think that women are not so much at risk for heart disease. We hear a lot about breast cancer and osteoporosis, but little about heart disease. In fact it is the number one killer of women — twice as many women die from heart disease as they do from all cancers combined.

It is after menopause that women become increasingly at risk. Unlike men, prior to this time we have had softer, more flexible arterial walls. One of the hormone-related changes at mid-life is a hardening of the arteries which, if we include the following risk factors, makes us as much at risk for heart disease, angina and heart attacks as men. Heart disease is associated with a refined food and high-fat diet, free-radical damage from smoking, stress, alcohol, environmental pollution, and sedentary lifestyles. Like other diseases, the incidence is much higher now than it used to be; in fact heart disease has reached epidemic proportions in Western countries. Heart disease is the primary cause of death of men and postmenopausal women in New Zealand, Australia, and the USA.

Our Western diet is particularly unbalanced with its excess of red meat and other foods high in saturated fats such as milk, cheese, ice cream and eggs. If you plot the incidence of heart attacks, atherosclerosis, breast cancer, and colon cancer in the world, the following countries will tend to fall to the bottom end for nearly every disease: Japan, Taiwan, Thailand, El Salvadore, and Sri Lanka. Others rise to the top: the United States, Canada, Australia, New Zealand, and Germany. If you chart the countries of the world according to how much milk, red meat, eggs, and cheese they consume, the same distribution will occur.

The underlying cause of cardiovascular disease is atherosclerosis — the thickening of blood vessel walls that leads to stiffness, brittleness and narrowing of the passageway. Atherosclerosis in arteries can progressively reduce the flow of blood, just as mineral deposits in a water pipe can block the flow of water.

Cholesterol has received a fair bit of bad press in relation to heart disease and particularly atherosclerosis. But it is not cholesterol levels that are the primary issue. Healthy cholesterol is in fact much needed by the body to produce hormones, bile acids, and cell membranes. The true nature of the problem has been narrowed down to first, a type of cholesterol known as low density lipoprotein (LDL), as opposed to high density lipoprotein (HDL — the 'good' cholesterol), and then to damaged LDL. Recent research has shown that atherosclerosis actually comes about not just as a result of high levels of LDL, but as a result of circulating LDL that has been attacked by oxygen or free radicals. This is called oxidised LDL or LDL-ox.

The body's own antioxidant defences against free radicals are varied and impressive, but they are not sufficient in themselves to maintain a steady state of good health, or prevent ageing or illness. Just as oxidation causes the formation of rust and the eventual breakdown of metal, slow motion oxidative stress is a reality for everyone. The free-radical clock is ticking!

A fundamental principle of Ayur-Vedic medicine is that nature provides an antidote or balancing factor for any imbalance that may occur. This certainly applies in the case of free radicals. Many naturally occurring foods have been found to contain substances that have antioxidant or free-radical-neutralising properties. These are the edible nutrients found in fruit and vegetables, nuts and seeds, which have been shown to quench free radicals, slow the ageing process and prevent serious degenerative diseases like heart disease and diabetes.

VITAMIN C

The most famous of the antioxidants is vitamin C. There is evidence now that vitamin C can add years to your life and that it offers protection to your arteries. It is a superb free-radical scavenger — particularly of the most reactive and lethal hydroxy radical. The human body cannot create its own vitamin C (although it was able to up to 250,000 years ago). Most animals do create their own, and when under stress they greatly increase their production of vitamin C — to fight the free radicals that stress creates.

Eating vitamin C rich foods and supplementing with modest amounts of vitamin C will protect against heart disease and cancer, and is effective in lowering blood pressure.[1]

An analysis of the diet of 11,000 Americans showed that women whose daily intake of vitamin C was around 300 mg daily (with roughly half of that as food) would live at least two years longer on average than those who had a low intake.[2] Good daily levels of vitamin C can increase 'good' HDL cholesterol levels, which in turn discourage clogging of the arteries and reduce 'bad' LDL cholesterol, which destroys arteries when it becomes oxidised from free-radical damage. This way, arteries stay flexible and younger. Vitamin C is a potent water-soluble antioxidant, which scavenges free radicals in the watery part of tissues. Vitamin E, on the other hand, is fat-soluble. The two work together to destroy free radicals.

Foods that are high in vitamin C are: citrus fruits and juices, sweet peppers, kiwifruit, strawberries, papaya, broccoli, Brussels sprouts, and tomatoes.

VITAMIN E

Vitamin E is found in the lipid membranes of the cell and acts as a first, fast-reacting defence against free-radical damage. Vitamin E actually enters the LDL molecule and sacrifices one of its own electrons (and thereby itself) to immobilise the free-radical oxygen molecule. The hypothesis that vitamin E can prevent cell membranes from oxidation caused by free-radical reactions was first advanced in 1983 and has since been proven correct by numerous credible scientific investigations. There is now general agreement that it is the most powerful of the antioxidants and it will prevent or reverse many degenerative diseases, including the greatest of them, atherosclerosis.

Several large-scale studies have shown that men and women who supplement with 100 IU/day of vitamin E for two or more years reduce their risk of fatal coronary heart disease and non-fatal heart attacks by 40 per cent. The researchers point out that the level of supplementation required for effective disease protection cannot be obtained through even the most well-balanced diet.[3] In 1993 researchers at the Harvard Medical School released a study showing that vitamin E supplementation prevents heart disease in women. Nurses who took more than 100 IU/day of vitamin E for more than two years reduced their risk of heart disease by 41 per cent.[4]

The benefits of an adequate vitamin E intake cannot be overemphasised. Unfortunately, to obtain a daily vitamin E intake of 400 IU it would be necessary to consume 200 cups of brown rice, 10 cups of almonds, 80 cups of cooked spinach or 12 tablespoons of unrefined, fresh wheatgerm oil! Supplementation is clearly necessary. The recommended daily intake of 400 IU of natural vitamin E combined with 250–1000 mg of vitamin C will help protect you against heart disease, cancer, and many other degenerative diseases.

Note: Natural vitamin E comes in several forms: d-alpha-tocopherol (100 mg = 149 IU), d-alpha-tocopherol acetate (100 mg = 136 IU), and d-alpha-tocopherol succinate are the most common. The 'd' designation in front indicates that the products are derived from natural sources such as vegetable oils or wheatgerm. A prefix of 'dl', such as dl-alpha-tocopherol, shows that the vitamin has been synthesised from a petroleum base. Synthetic vitamin E is far less effective than natural vitamin E.

BETA-CAROTENE

A third micronutrient, beta-carotene, has been researched in addition to vitamins C and E. Beta-carotene is the substance that gives carrots their colour. It is a precursor to vitamin A as the body converts it to vitamin A in the small intestine. Beta-carotene works effectively against free radicals and has a well-documented ability to fight cancer.[5] (Note: beta-carotene is one of a large group of carotenoids. It is best to take a complex of carotenoids.)

COENZYME Q10

Coenzyme Q10 or ubiquinol is a natural substance produced by your body. We tend to become deficient in it as we age. It is being hailed as one of the most important and effective antioxidants for preventing the oxidation of LDL and thereby atherosclerosis. Several studies have shown that patients with congestive heart failure and other cardiovascular diseases have significantly lower levels of coenzyme Q10 in their heart tissue than healthy people. Supplementation with as little as 100 mg per day has been shown to improve the condition remarkably.[6]

VITAMIN B_6 AND FOLIC ACID

A very recent major study from the Harvard School of Public Health shows that a higher intake of folic acid and vitamin B_6 (pyridoxine) protects women against non-fatal and fatal coronary heart disease. The study followed the dietary habits of 80,000 female nurses from 1980 to 1994. Statistical analysis showed that women whose intake of folate (folic acid) exceeded 545 micrograms/day had a 31 per cent lower risk of having a heart attack or fatal coronary heart disease than did women whose intake was less than 153 micrograms per day. Similarly, women whose intake of vitamin B_6 was greater than 5.9 milligrams per day had a 33 per cent lower risk. Women with the highest intake of both folate and vitamin B_6 had a 45 per cent lower risk than women with the lowest combined intake. These risk reductions were independent of other heart disease risk factors such as smoking, hypertension, alcohol consumption, and the intake of fibre, vitamin E and saturated, polyunsaturated and trans fatty acids. Most of the women used multivitamins and other vitamin supplements for their daily intake of folate and vitamin B_6.[7,8]

VITAMIN B_3 (NIACIN)

In a very recent study of patients diagnosed with vascular disease, the researchers concluded that niacin supplementation is effective in lowering fibrinogen and LDL levels while at the same time increasing the level of HDL.[9]

AMRIT KALASH

Many studies of an ancient Ayur-Vedic formula called Amrit Kalash have revealed that the most effective free-radical scavenger of them all comes from the world's oldest system of health care. The recipes for these ancient formulations of fruits and herbs were first discovered thousands of years ago, and the knowledge, though largely lost to the public, was guarded by a small number of custodians and passed down over time through the generations. Results of studies at the Niwa Institute in Japan and at research institutes in the USA into the effects of Amrit Kalash on the human immune system have shown that it is as effective as the body's own antioxidant enzyme superoxide dismutase in scavenging the 'master' free-radical superoxide.[10,11] Repeated clinical trials have revealed it to be an antioxidant that is literally one thousand times more effective than vitamin E or vitamin C.[12] (See Resources, page 224.)

HIGH BLOOD PRESSURE

Calcium, potassium and magnesium are important. A four-year study of 60,000 nurses concluded that women who have a calcium intake of 800 mg per day or more have a 23 per cent lower risk of developing high blood pressure than women with an intake of 400 mg per day or less.[13]

The effect of potassium on high blood pressure is still being actively investigated. One trial found that a 50 per cent increase in potassium from natural foods lowered blood pressure and dramatically reduced the need for blood pressure lowering drugs.

Several studies suggest that a low magnesium intake is associated with hypertension, stroke, and ischemic heart disease. It has been proposed that supplementation with about 900 mg per day of magnesium is required in order to effectively lower blood pressure.[14]

DAILY DIET

Be aware of the dangers of eating processed foods — particularly if they include hydrogenated oils or polyunsaturated oils which are almost certain to have been processed in some way; even if they haven't been, they will probably be rancid. Use olive oil for cooking. Mediterranean cultures, famous for their lavish use of olive oil, are remarkably free of heart disease and some forms of cancer even though they have a high total fat intake.[15]

Overall, reduce your intake of fats and oils. We need such a small amount each day. Eat only minimal amounts of butter and saturated fat. Favour eating fresh vegetables, fruits, seeds and nuts as a source of essential polyunsaturated fats.

As a general rule, most plants are richly endowed with antioxidants. Bioflavanoids are the natural substances that create the beautiful deep blues and reds in fruits, berries and wine. They are effective free-radical scavengers known to slow the development of heart disease and be effective against cancer, and to reduce allergies and asthma.

HRT

Women who are found to be at risk for heart disease have been encouraged to take hormone replacement therapy. However, a recent clinical trial examining the role of HRT in treating women with established heart disease reveals that it may not be beneficial. In fact HRT appears to increase the risk of heart attacks and gallbladder disease.[16]

STRESS

Physical health and psychological health go hand in hand. Modern medicine has recently found objective evidence to support what we all instinctively know — feeling good can make you well! A recent study involving 132 patients who already had coronary artery disease concluded that moderate to strong feelings of sadness, tension, and frustration could more than double the risk of these patients having a myocardial ischemia event (heart attack).[17]

Another study found that men who worried a lot about the world situation and social conditions had a 50 per cent greater risk of developing any form of heart disease than men who never or rarely worried.[18]

Chronic stress results in constant free-radical generation. This means that effective stress management should slow the creation of excess free radicals, and significantly improve our health. Once again, studies show that people practising TM have much lower risk for stress-related diseases. A comparative study measuring 2000 people practising TM found that the TM group had 87 per cent less hospitalisation for heart disease.[19]

EXERCISE

No group is at higher risk for depression, disease and early death than people who are completely sedentary. Exercise is essential for overall health and has been shown to reduce risk factors for heart disease like high blood pressure, help prevent osteoporosis, and improve blood sugar tolerance. It is also fun and a wonderful addition to the daily routine. Walking is a great way to exercise. A recent study of elderly retired men in the US showed that regular walking increases longevity and that the risk of death can be reduced by 19 per cent for every one mile increase in daily walking distance.[20] A new study shows that exercise is necessary if you are on a low-fat diet to normalise cholesterol levels. Diet alone will not reduce 'bad' cholesterol levels whereas according to the study, the addition of exercise will reduce them by 15–20 per cent.[21]

SUMMARY

Factors known to reduce the risk for heart disease:
- Minimising free-radical damage by increasing your daily intake of antioxidants
- Controlling high blood pressure
- Having a good diet — avoiding too much saturated fat and trans fatty acids and eating LOTS of fresh fruits, vegetables, nuts and seeds
- Avoiding smoking
- Avoiding alcohol
- Exercising regularly
- Lowering stress levels through lifestyle changes and meditation
- Inadequate mineral intake

10
DEPRESSION AT MID-LIFE

Happiness depends upon ourselves.
Aristotle

Women at menopause are less likely to be depressed than younger women. In New Zealand, depression is most common in women in their early thirties. But there are exceptions. Those who have had a history of depression, who have a low income, have experienced stressful life events such as bereavement, and have a negative view of menopause are more likely to be depressed. It has been found that women who expect that menopause will bring a host of physical and emotional problems do tend to be more affected by it.[1,2,3]

Research has dismissed the link between hormonal changes and depression at mid-life and suggests that additional life stresses at this time are more likely to be the cause of poor psychological health than menopause itself.[4] Caring for elderly relatives, for example, can be very stressful — approximately 25 per cent of women have this responsibility at menopause. It can also coincide with children leaving home, job responsibilities, and career or primary relationship upheaval.

In her excellent book *Women's Bodies, Women's Wisdom*,

DEPRESSION AT MID-LIFE

Christiane Northrup comments on Sonja McKinlay's research of healthy menopausal women who were not seeking medical advice. Her study revealed that for the majority of women, menopause is not the major negative event it has been typified as. 'One unique feature of this study is that it was done on healthy women ... clearly, many physicians have a negative view of menopause based on their biased population.'

She does acknowledge, however, that it is hard for some women. 'Menopause is a time when we are preparing to move into our wisdom years, and we may come up against the "unfinished business" that we have accumulated over the first half of our life. We may find ourselves grieving for losses never fully grieved, longing to get a college degree that we never completed, or longing for another child or a first child. All the unfinished business of women's lives comes up at menopause to be reexamined and completed, as if we have gone down into our basement and found boxes and boxes of stuff to be sorted and weeded out.' She goes on to say that when a woman is willing to resolve the unfinished business of her life, no treatment of her mood swings is necessary.[5]

That aside, many of us do suffer from mild depression, anxiety, exhaustion or the 'blues' sometimes without even realising it. Many things affect mood. In the winter, it is common to feel more sleepy and sad and to gain weight. This is a malaise that has the name 'seasonal affective disorder' (or SAD) and women are apparently twice as likely to be afflicted by it. Exercise and a walk in the sun can often be all that is required to lift the spirits, and the symptoms are usually temporary.

PHYSICAL CAUSE OF DEPRESSION

Surgical removal of the uterus (hysterectomy) can be a cause of depression for some women. In a 1997 study involving 285 women who had had a hysterectomy, paired with a control group of women who had not, it was found that depression was more frequent among those women who had had a hysterectomy.[6]

Recent studies have shown that as many as 10 per cent of all women over 60 years of age could have problems relating to thyroid dysfunction. Dr Kenneth Woeber, MD of the University of California, recommends that women older than 60 years who suffer from major depression could be suffering from thyroid conditions and should undergo the appropriate tests.[7]

There is some evidence that people with dental amalgam fillings containing mercury are more likely to suffer from depression than people without such fillings. In a study of patients suffering from manic depression (bi-polar disorder), the removal of amalgam from their teeth resulted in very significant improvement in anxiety levels, depression, paranoia, hostility, and obsessive-compulsive behaviour.[8] (Other studies have shown that amalgam fillings may also be a significant factor in hearing loss.[9])

WHAT IS DEPRESSION?

Depression is more than just the occasional bad mood. It is a medical illness with recognisable symptoms. In the USA it has reached epidemic proportions where it is estimated that 21,000 suicides annually are the direct result of untreated depression. It is the number one cause of alcoholism, drug abuse, eating disorders, and other addictions. A significant number of divorces, spousal and child abuse, absenteeism from work, lost jobs, and bankruptcies are attributed to depression. Neither are we immune to it. Approximately one million antidepressants were dispensed in New Zealand in the last financial year.

In his recent book *Hypericum and Depression*, Harold Bloomfield lists the following symptoms of depression:

- Persistent sad or 'empty' mood
- Loss of pleasure in ordinary activities, including sex
- Decreased energy, fatigue, being 'slowed down'
- Sleep disturbances (insomnia, early-morning wakening, or oversleeping)
- Eating disturbances (loss of appetite and weight, or weight gain)

DEPRESSION AT MID-LIFE

- Feelings of guilt, worthlessness, helplessness
- Thoughts of death or suicide, suicide attempts
- Irritability
- Excessive crying
- Chronic aches and pains that don't respond to treatment

In the workplace, the symptoms of depression often may be recognised by:

- Decreased productivity
- Morale problems
- Lack of cooperation
- Safety problems, accidents
- Absenteeism
- Frequent complaints of being tired all the time
- Complaints of unexplained aches and pains
- Alcohol and drug abuse[10]

Major depression is described as either mild, moderate, or severe. The vast majority of major depressions fall in the mild-to-moderate range.

ST JOHN'S WORT

If you suffer from mild to moderate depression, you may find it helpful to take *Hypericum* or St John's wort. There is now a wealth of evidence that it can help overcome depression and anxiety, and have a levelling effect on the emotions. St John's wort is currently the most extensively researched and used herbal antidepressant. It has an excellent safety record too. After centuries of recorded use in Europe and extensive recent use in Germany there are no medical reports of toxicity or serious drug reactions. It has no sedative effect and it does not react with alcohol.

ANCIENT RECORDED USE

St John's wort has featured as a herbal medicine since ancient times. Dioscorides, the foremost physician of ancient Greece, as well as Pliny in ancient Rome, administered St John's wort in the treatment of many illnesses. Its main use was to treat wounds, nervous conditions, fluid retention, sciatica, kidney and lung ailments, and malaria.

Hippocrates, the father of medicine, and the medical herbalist Galen wrote about the medicinal properties of St John's wort and there are significant writings of its use spanning the centuries.[11] It was believed that the plant was a powerful repellent for warding off evil spirits, that a whiff of it would cause them to fly away. Early Christians would tie pieces of the plant over doorways or around the neck, or would place pieces under a pillow to dispel evil and bring good luck. In England and Europe, the belief in *Hypericum*'s magical properties continued from ancient times to the Middle Ages.

BOTANICAL INFORMATION

The botanical name is *Hypericum perforatum* — based on the perforated appearance of the leaf glands when held up to the light. A beautiful perennial plant, it grows freely in the wild to 30cm to 1m tall and produces bright yellow flowers about 4cm in diameter with five petals. The petals have numerous black dots containing a red pigment. *Hypericum* flowers around the summer solstice in the Northern Hemisphere — a possible reason for the name as it coincides with St John (the Baptist's) Day on 24 June. It is thought that the red, oil-filled spots on the plant's leaves were symbolic of the saint's blood and were thought to appear on or around the anniversary of his beheading. In New Zealand and Australia the flowers first appear in November and flowering continues well into summer.

In New Zealand, St John's wort is officially a plant pest, being one of more than 100 plants named in the National Surveillance Plant Pests list. You cannot legally propagate, distribute or sell the plant in New Zealand, although you can sell products made from it. It is banned because of its potential to damage native ecosystems and because of phototoxicity (light sensitivity) in animals that have grazed heavily on it. Light-skinned animals such as sheep may die from exposure to sun after ingesting large quantities. St John's wort increases their susceptibility to sunlight and they can actually die from extreme sunburn. Not one case of phototoxicity has been documented in humans at depression dosages, or even after accidental overdose.

The actions of St John's wort have been recorded as sedative, astringent and diuretic, and useful for nervous affectations with depression, haemorrhages, diarrhoea and chronic urinary tract problems. It is specific for spinal injuries and is used externally for bruises, wounds, ulcers and tumours. It is also recommended for bed-wetting and night terrors in children. It has been used topically as a mild analgesic. Recent interest has focused on its possible role as an antiviral agent. Its recent popularity is as a side-effect and risk-free antidepressant. It is reported to be safer to use than aspirin — there have been no reported deaths in over 2400 years of use.

Physicians in Germany routinely prescribe herbal medicines, and St John's wort is used widely as an antidepressant. In 1994 six million doses of *Hypericum* were prescribed for the treatment of depression, accounting for sales of over $US50 million. Today 20 million people are reported to be taking it regularly, its sales outnumbering Prozac 25–1. In New Zealand, following a *20/20* programme in 1997, sales of St John's wort in health food stores went from minimal to very high overnight. Within 24 hours, Auckland was sold out!

Paula was one of the people who started using St John's wort at this time. 'I began taking St John's wort after seeing the TV programme. Basically, I tried it as a last resort for my severe insomnia, which had failed to respond to every other herbal or over-the-counter-treatment. Its effect was simply amazing. The very day I took St John's wort, I had the first full, restful night of sleep in over six months. And I have slept all night long, every night since. I could not believe it could work so fast, or so well. I have had no side-effects at all. Rather, a startling change in my emotional state has taken place. I had been suffering from a mild depression characterised by severe emotional highs and lows — and I did not even fully realise what was happening until it was gone. I have become a pleasant, happy person! My constant anxieties have disappeared. My husband is overjoyed that my irritability and moodiness have at last gone away.'

WHAT IS IN ST JOHN'S WORT?

St John's wort contains many compounds that are known to be biologically active. It is believed that the effectiveness of the herb lies in the combination of the variety of active ingredients rather than any single one. The constituents hypericin and pseudo-hypericin are the two that are considered to be essential or most important for many of the known effects. The extract also contains flavanoids such as quercetin, xanthones, and bioflavanoids. The red-coloured hypericins have been found in very few other plants while most of *Hypericum*'s other ingredients are common in the plant kingdom.

The active ingredients are obtained through alcohol extraction — the flowering and leafy portions of the plant are dried, and alcohol is used to dissolve the useful elements of the plant. When the alcohol evaporates, the extract remains leaving no alcohol in the finished product. The plant chemicals also dissolve well in oil. The plant has to be air dried in the shade away from light in order to protect the photosensitive active ingredients.

BENEFITS CONFIRMED BY RECENT RESEARCH

A team of German and American researchers evaluated the results of 23 randomised trials on the effectiveness of St John's wort as an antidepressant. The studies involved over 1750 patients with mild to moderate depression. The research published in the *British Medical Journal* in 1996 concluded that *Hypericum* is almost three times as effective as a placebo and equally effective as commonly used antidepressants, without side-effects such as headaches or vomiting. From 50–80 per cent of people suffering from depression received relief, increased appetite, more interest in life, greater self-esteem and restoration of normal sleeping patterns.

The researchers concluded that *Hypericum* is effective in treating certain types of depression, but that longer-term studies are necessary to determine whether it is effective in treating severe depression and whether some preparations are more effective than others. 'St John's wort is a promising treatment for depression ... *Hypericum* extracts were significantly superior to placebo and similarly effective as standard antidepressants. The herb may offer an advantage, however, in terms of relative safety and tolerability, which might improve patient compliance.'[12, 13]

Over the coming years, any unanswered questions about *Hypericum*'s effectiveness and safety may finally be settled. A new major clinical trial by the National Institute of Health (NIH) in the US is now underway to fully measure *Hypericum*'s effectiveness in the treatment of depression. The trial will involve 366 patients diagnosed with a moderate form of depression. Each participant will be randomly treated with one of three options — a uniform dose of *Hypericum*, a placebo, or a selective seratonin uptake inhibitor (like Prozac). A standardised preparation containing a 900 mg daily dose of *Hypericum* will be used in the study. This will be the first large and long-term study to fully assess the therapeutic value of *Hypericum*.[14]

It has been discovered recently that St John's wort is active against viruses and is now also used to treat certain kinds of viral infections. Research is underway to assess its potential action against retroviruses including the big one, HIV — the virus that causes AIDS.

HOW DOES IT WORK?

Many of today's antidepressant medications work by inhibiting the enzyme mono-amine oxidase, which slows down the breakdown of the neurotransmitters norepinephrine and seratonin, increasing their concentration in the central nervous system. These transmitters are responsible for maintaining emotional stability and mood.

Other antidepressants such as Prozac work by affecting the uptake of seratonin, thereby increasing its concentration in the central nervous system. Although it is not fully understood how it works, St John's wort appears to have both these actions, which could be why some claim it manages depression better than other prescribed forms of treatment.

Hypericin, one of the active ingredients in St John's wort, has been found to accumulate in the brain, stomach and skin tissue, but is more rapidly excreted in other tissues. This may explain why its main site of action seems to be in the brain, and why there are minimal side-effects.

WHAT ARE THE SIDE-EFFECTS AND CONTRAINDICATIONS?

Only 2.4 per cent of people involved in studies of St John's wort have experienced side-effects, and these have been minimal: 0.5 per cent experienced allergic reactions, 0.4 per cent tiredness/fatigue and 0.3 per cent restlessness.

On the positive side, any side-effects will go away as soon as a person stops taking St John's wort. The *British Medical Journal* study concluded that side-effects were 'rare and mild'. Studies have shown that St John's wort does not affect the ability to think or to drive. It has been shown to have a long-term effect on anxiety comparable to Valium, without the side-effects.

If you are not taking any antidepressant drug, then St John's wort is perfectly safe to take. You should, however, consult a herbalist for exact instructions. St John's wort takes two to six weeks to take full effect. If you are already using a pharmaceutical antidepressant for mild to moderate depression and you want to try St John's wort then consult your doctor and a professional herbalist. St John's wort is not sufficient for people with severe depression, although one study has shown promising results. In the meantime, if you are suffering from severe depression you need to be under the care of a health professional, and may do better with prescription antidepressants.

Not a lot is known about taking St John's wort with prescription antidepressants or switching from one to the other. Therefore it is strongly recommended that this is done only with professional help. It is not advisable to suddenly stop taking prescription antidepressants as this can result in severe 'rebound' depression. St John's wort is not intended to replace lithium, tricyclics, and specific panic/anxiety drugs.

St John's wort is best avoided if you are pregnant or breastfeeding. It is possible that it could affect breast milk production, as it is known to inhibit secretion of the milk-producing hormone prolactin.

RECOMMENDED DOSES OF ST JOHN'S WORT

The optimum recommended dose based on current knowledge and research is 300 mg of *Hypericum* extract three times a day — that is, a total of 900 mg spread throughout the day. You can work out the best times to take it through trial and error. If you have difficulty sleeping you may want to save the final dose for dinner or bedtime. Because *Hypericum* is well tolerated by the body it is believed that little harm can come from experimenting with dosages, as side-effects are few even in significantly higher doses. It is recommended that six full weeks at the full dose elapse before results of effectiveness are evaluated.

The herb is sold in different forms. Some common doses include:

- One 300 mg capsule three times a day
- 30 to 40 drops of oil mixed in water, two to five times a day
- One to two teaspoons of the dried herb added to boiling water, then steeped for 15 minutes before drinking, three times per day

Small children should take a total of 300 mg daily and larger children 600 mg.

SOME SUCCESS STORIES

1. *'I had been mildly depressed for most of my life, and wouldn't even know anything was wrong — except that I had a period of my life a few years back when my depression spontaneously disappeared for about a year. Then I got knocked into a bout of major depression (which I am just coming out of) which prompted my research into treatment options.*

'My current self-medication regime includes a dietary modification [of reduced sugar and carbohydrate intake] and St John's wort — and it is working. At three months I am no longer depressed, I have regained the capacity for taking pleasure in life, and I have regained a sense of connection to the people around me, and to the world in general, and the ability to anticipate pleasure and joy. I have regained my libido, and sex is once again the joy I believe it should be. I am physically feeling much better, have much more energy, and I am no longer prone to all the little colds and infections that I used to get. I am interested in things again, and I no longer feel like I couldn't be bothered living. Life IS worth living, and there IS joy in the world.'

2. *'I am a nurse who is well aware of the different antidepressants out there, their side-effects etc . . . As long as I can remember I have always had this overwhelming feeling of sadness, but could never quite place a finger on why. In the early eighties I was placed on a prescription antidepressant, but because of the side-effects only took it for a couple of weeks. I never took anything after that, and suffered through many bouts of "depression", having semi-frequent suicidal thoughts. I believe my depression is somewhat responsible for my failed relationships in life. I started using St John's wort about one and a half months ago, taking only two 250 mg capsules per day. After two to three weeks all of a sudden I felt great! I was ecstatic, no more sad feelings or suicidal thoughts. It is truly remarkable.'*

3. *'I am one of those for whom taking St John's wort "did the trick". I had been told by various people over the years that I should be "on something" for depression, but I did not feel comfortable taking any kind of prescription drug, especially one which would alter my mood. However, when I saw an article in Newsweek about St John's wort and it specifically said that it has been prescribed for people who do not feel comfortable on prescription medication, I had felt so rotten for so long that I thought I would give it a try. I did not expect it to work, so I was quite shocked when, in a matter of DAYS, not weeks as the article had stated, I felt GREAT! For the first time in my life I felt like I was going to be OK no matter what. My thoughts of suicide went away, and I found it easier to let go of situations I could do nothing about. I feel more at ease in social situations, and much more confident. I had not realised how serious my depression was until it was gone. Now I only feel bad when something happens that would make most people feel that way. It has been an amazing transformation. I have never taken an antidepressant, and I don't even really believe in "herbal medicine", but I'm going to take this stuff forever if I have to. So I'll just stick with it, and be grateful that my stubborn resistance to taking drugs didn't keep me from trying this. It has really changed my life.'*

Disclaimer: 'Natural' substances can have harmful side-effects, especially if taken with other substances, or in large quantities. As St John's wort is not a proven therapy for depression, there is some risk in using it. Clinical depression is a serious medical disorder that can be debilitating and can lead to suicide. Currently the effective, proven treatments are antidepressants, short-term specific psychotherapies, or a combination of both. Since other medical conditions, such as thyroid disorders, can also mimic depression, anyone with symptoms of depression should receive a thorough medical examination to rule out other possible causes of the symptoms. If you are taking any heart medication, please consult your doctor before taking St John's wort.

TREATMENTS FOR ANXIETY

KAVA KAVA
Piper methysticum

Kava kava as a treatment for anxiety and mood swings has recently become popular. It is possible to purchase products that contain both St John's wort and kava kava.

Kava kava, a member of the pepper family, is one of the most fascinating of medicinal plants. It is native to the South Pacific, and a beverage (also called kava) made from the rootstock of the plant has been used for centuries in ceremonies and celebrations because of its calming effect and ability to promote sociability. The kava beverage is still used today by the island communities of the Pacific.

Explorer Captain James Cook gave the plant the botanical name of *Piper methysticum* — intoxicating pepper. Kava kava has been used for over 3000 years for its medicinal effects as a sedative, muscle relaxant, diuretic, and as a remedy for nervousness and insomnia.

Kava kava is now recognised as an excellent treatment and alternative to tranquillisers in the treatment of anxiety. In Germany, it is used as a non-prescription drug to reduce anxiety. Kava kava was first mentioned in scientific records in 1886, and is gaining popularity in the US for its relaxing effects.

Studies have shown that long-term use lowers nervous anxiety, tension and restlessness after eight weeks.[15] German researchers have conducted five well-designed studies on more than 400 subjects since 1990 and all subjects have had positive results from their careful and monitored use of kava kava extracts.

Clinical studies have shown that the herb is a safe, non-addictive, anti-anxiety medicine, and as effective as prescription anti-anxiety agents containing benzodiazepines, such as Valium. While benzodiazepines tend to promote lethargy and mental impairment, kava kava has been clinically demonstrated as a means of achieving a state of relaxation without the adverse side-effects. The plant works by first stimulating the nervous system, and then depressing it.

Contraindications

Because it is a powerful herb, some guidelines are in order. Seek the advice of a health professional and always go by the recommended dose. Botanical specialists do not recommend kava kava for clinical depressive disorders, either mild or more serious. It's not that kava kava will harm patients with such disorders, it just hasn't been shown to help them. They also caution against mixing kava kava with other anti-anxiety prescriptions or alcohol, as kava kava may intensify their actions. In addition, some caution that dopamine levels may be affected by kava kava and advise that it should be avoided by those with Parkinson's disease. They also caution against use by pregnant or lactating women or in combination with alcoholic beverages. Consult your physician if you are taking other medications such as benzodiazepine tranquillisers.

OTHER TREATMENTS FOR ANXIETY

In a large exhaustive study published in the *Journal of Clinical Psychology*, nearly two decades of stress-related studies and various meditation and relaxation techniques were compared statistically. In the results of all the tests together, Transcendental Meditation was shown to reduce anxiety twice as much as any other technique.[16]

Black cohosh, the traditional herb typically prescribed for menopause, is calming, and has been shown to be helpful for mood swings, anxiety and depression when combined with St John's wort.[17]

11
MINERALS

Minerals are the basic building blocks of good health. The body needs at least 60 different minerals every day in food and water to perform its functions properly and maintain a healthy immune system. Plants are able to manufacture vitamins, but they cannot manufacture minerals, so they take up and consequently remove available minerals from the soil as they grow. Our soils have become depleted of minerals from years of agriculture, heavy cropping and erosion. Low soil mineral content means that our food in turn has much lower levels of the minerals essential for our bodies, such as calcium, magnesium, boron, manganese, selenium and chromium.

Quite apart from soil depletion, it is difficult to get the full quota of minerals from locally grown food. The 60 or so minerals that are essential to us are not distributed in an even blanket over the surface of the Earth — they tend to occur naturally in veins of varying amounts from place to place. In New Zealand our soils are deficient in the trace minerals zinc, selenium and iodine.

Minerals can be thought of as the source of life, and are so important for normal functioning that the body may go to desperate lengths to maintain their balance. For example, calcium is essential for normal growth and development. If the body is deficient in calcium, it may take calcium out of the bones in an attempt to make up the deficiency.

It is not only the quantity of minerals that is important — their ratios to each other are also important. Two or more minerals often work in conjunction with each other at the cellular level. An example is the interaction of the minerals sodium and potassium, which enable cells to take in nutrients and dispose of waste material. If the two minerals are not correctly balanced, cells will be either undernourished or they will drown in their own waste material.

As a further illustration, most of us learn that to avoid osteoporosis, we must take plenty of calcium. That's a good start, but many of us don't realise that calcium is not absorbed properly without the correct amounts of the minerals magnesium and boron, and the vitamins A, C and D.

The trace mineral selenium, largely missing from New Zealand soil, is a powerful antioxidant and is an essential step in the body's production of glutathione peroxidase, an enzyme that neutralises free radicals. When selenium levels in soils have been plotted geographically throughout the world, cancer levels have been found to be higher in those areas that have low levels of selenium.[1] Studies in the US have shown that selenium supplementation helps prevent cancer and appears to inhibit the growth of tumours.[2,3]

Plants take up through their root systems whatever minerals are in the soil, so the amount of minerals in crops depends on exactly where they are grown. All of the minerals that crops take up from the soil are removed with the plants at each harvest. Farmers are encouraged to produce the most crops for the lowest cost, and they learned long ago that they only need to add three minerals to the soil — nitrogen, phosphorus and potassium (NPK) — to produce the maximum growth.

After a few years of farming this way, with every available mineral being taken up and only three being replaced, the soil has been gradually depleted of most of the trace minerals, so crops no longer contain sufficient quantities of the 60 minerals that we need to function properly. Unless farmers added NPK to the soil each year, there would not be enough minerals in the soil to produce any crops at all, let alone nutritionally rich crops.

The remaining minerals are replenished only if the soil is irrigated by water that is rich in minerals. For example, the land adjacent to the river Nile in Egypt used to produce mineral-rich crops every year because it was irrigated every spring by the flood waters, which were rich in minerals from their turbulent passage through the mountains of Ethiopia. Unfortunately, today the river flow is controlled and most food is produced from farmland that is irrigated by river water that is not rich in minerals. Soils have historically been remineralised during ice ages. Increasing agricultural demands on the land and an ever-increasing world population calls for urgent intensive full re-mineralisation of soils by farmers.

To make matters more serious, many minerals are lost from food during processing at commercial food-refining and processing plants. The following are the percentage losses of some minerals through the refinement of flour in New Zealand:

Calcium	66 per cent
Magnesium	66 per cent
Chromium	80 per cent (approx)
Manganese	86 per cent
Zinc	77 per cent

The trace mineral chromium is necessary for the proper metabolism of all forms of sugar — natural and processed. Today, practically all processed foods contain sugar, yet the staple food, flour, loses much of the chromium necessary to process that sugar. This increases the risk of glucose intolerance and diabetes, and is thought to be partly responsible for attention deficiency disorders.

As long ago as 1936, US scientists found soils to be seriously deficient because of cropping and pollution. The 1936 United States Senate Document 264, published by the second session of the 74th Congress stated:

> 'Most of us today are suffering from certain dangerous diet deficiencies which cannot be remedied until the depleted soils from which our foods come are brought into proper mineral balance.
>
> 'The alarming fact is that foods — fruits, vegetables and grains now being raised on millions of acres of land that no longer contain enough of certain minerals — are starving us, no matter how much of them we eat!
>
> 'You'd think, wouldn't you, that a carrot is a carrot — that one is about as good as another as far as nourishment is concerned? But it isn't; one carrot may look and taste like another and yet be lacking in the particular mineral element which our system requires and which carrots are supposed to contain.
>
> 'Laboratory tests prove that the fruits, the vegetables, the grains, the eggs, and even the milk and the meats of today are not what they were a few generations ago (which doubtless explains why our forefathers thrived on a selection of foods that would starve us!).
>
> 'No man of today can eat enough fruits and vegetables to supply his stomach with the mineral salts he requires for perfect health because his stomach isn't big enough to hold them!
>
> 'It is bad news to learn from our leading authorities that 99 per cent of the American people are deficient in these minerals, and that a marked deficiency in any one of the more important minerals actually results in disease. Any upset of the balance, any considerable lack of one or another element, however microscopic the body requirement may be, and we sicken, suffer, and shorten our lives.
>
> 'Lacking vitamins, the system can make some use of minerals, but lacking minerals, vitamins are useless.'

Nearly 60 years later, the 1992 Rio Earth Summit Report

summarised the percentage depletion of soil minerals over the last 100 years as follows:

North America	85 per cent
South America	76 per cent
Asia	76 per cent
Africa	74 per cent
Europe	72 per cent
Australia	55 per cent

ESSENTIAL MINERALS

The list of trace minerals essential for human health is growing. It now includes zinc, copper, manganese, iron, molybdenum, selenium, chromium, nickel, silicon, arsenic, lithium and boron. The best available method of determining what minerals you are lacking is hair mineral analysis which identifies any deficiencies by giving you a read-out of your levels of all the major minerals (see Resources, page 224). The majority of trace minerals do not show up in blood tests. It may be necessary to take dietary supplements in order to get your daily mineral requirement. A lack of complete knowledge has led researchers to caution about single mineral supplementation, however. Extensive work is underway to determine the safe and desirable intake range, but in the meantime purchase balanced mineral supplements and avoid excessive doses. For maximum absorption minerals should be in a plant-derived colloidal form.

Soils can be re-mineralised through the topical application of balanced minerals onto the land. We can do this in our own gardens and grow vegetables this way, or we can try to buy organic fruit and vegetables grown in re-mineralised soils (see Resources, page 224).

MAGNESIUM

Magnesium is involved in the functioning of more than 200 enzymes and is a key player in the body's energy cycle. Magnesium is a 'master' mineral that coordinates the proper functioning of nerves, muscle, blood vessels and bone. Magnesium deficiency is widespread in New Zealand with the average intake being more than 20 per cent below the daily recommended level of 300mg. The body's requirement for magnesium is increased markedly by both stress and vigorous exercise. Magnesium is essential for energy production, and even a slight deficiency could account for low energy levels. It is known that exercise capacity can be significantly increased by the use of magnesium supplements.

Magnesium has a relaxing effect and has been used in the treatment of anxiety disorders. It can also help with PMS symptoms like breast tenderness, and with migraine.

Magnesium is found in sea vegetables, whole grains, nuts, seeds and legumes. Nuts are one of the richest sources of magnesium — particularly almonds, hazelnuts, cashews, pine nuts, peanuts, walnuts, and pecans.

Magnesium deficiency is often implicated in heart disease. A 1997 study in northern India with a total of 3575 subjects aged 25–63 years showed that men and women with a low consumption of dietary magnesium had a higher prevalence of coronary artery disease and of the coronary risk factors hypertension, high cholesterol, and diabetes.[4] Researchers in the US at the University Medical Centre in Tucson have confirmed that magnesium deficiency is closely associated with heart disease. Lowered levels of magnesium in the blood have been found in heart-attack patients, and injections of magnesium following heart attacks have been found to reduce mortality rate by 24 per cent.[5,6,7]

MAGNESIUM AND BONES

Many researchers are now reporting that magnesium deficiency plays a big part in the development of osteoporosis. Studies have shown that women suffering from osteoporosis tend to have a lower magnesium intake than normal, and also have lower levels of magnesium in their bones. It is also clear that calcium must be taken with magnesium for optimum effect, and that a magnesium deficiency can affect the production of vitamin D, further risking osteoporosis. The recommended ratio of calcium to magnesium is 2:1.

Some studies show that magnesium supplementation *alone* is effective in treating osteoporosis — that it can prevent further bone loss, and in some cases can even increase bone density. A Czechoslovakian study showed that women who supplemented daily with 1500 to 3000mg of magnesium for two years were rid of their pain and stopped further development of deformities of the vertebrae.[8] If you think you are not getting enough magnesium from food, take a supplement of 200 to 300mg. A chelated form is best (bound with protein for better absorption).

If you have kidney problems or heart failure, consult your doctor before taking magnesium supplements.

ZINC

Zinc is an essential mineral that can be found in all body tissues, but especially in the eye, liver, brain, muscle, and reproductive organs. A deficiency in zinc puts you at risk of infections, as it strengthens immune system function. There are indicators that many individuals are zinc deficient once they reach mid-life because of poor eating habits, and because the ability to absorb zinc lessens as we age.[9] The recommended daily amount is difficult to achieve as food refinement takes out valuable zinc from many of our grains. A high-fibre diet can reduce effective absorption of zinc. Vegetarians are likely to be low in zinc because it is found mostly in meat and poultry. The best sources of zinc are raw oysters and lean meats. Cereals, nuts and seeds are relatively high in zinc, but they also contain agents that reduce zinc absorption.

A zinc deficiency can lead to problems with wound healing, reduced immune function, loss of taste and smell and reduced levels of testosterone in the blood. For many older people a mild zinc deficiency could put them at a higher risk of infections and the degenerative diseases of ageing.[10] Short-term ingestion of zinc has been found to substantially reduce the severity of a cold.[11]

Modest amounts of zinc supplementation (up to 9mg) daily have been found to correct deficiencies and boost immunity. The most absorbable forms of zinc are zinc gluconate or zinc citrate. An excessive intake of zinc can lead to a copper deficiency. Recent experiments have confirmed this finding and researchers calculate that supplementing with more than 9mg per day of zinc may be unsafe.[12] It is best to get a doctor's advice if any more than this is taken.

A study of elderly women found that those taking calcium supplementation reduced their zinc absorption. Therefore those following recommendations to substantially increase their calcium intake to prevent bone loss may need to further supplement their zinc intake with 10mg daily (only about 20 per cent of ingested zinc is absorbed by the body).[13]

CHROMIUM

The single overriding reason to take chromium is to prevent having too much of the hormone insulin in your blood. As we age, our cells become less efficient at using insulin to process blood sugar. This results in an excess of insulin in the bloodstream. The dangers of this are that it can advance to a diabetic condition, but before that it can mean that high blood sugar can increase levels of LDL cholesterol and triglycerides, therefore directly increasing the risk of heart disease. Chromium helps prevent an insulin imbalance by optimising insulin activity, and if you lack chromium, your insulin and blood sugar levels will increase. Heart patients have been found to have low levels of chromium in their blood — up to 40 per cent lower than healthy individuals.[14] Pioneering research carried out by the US Department of Agriculture has emphasised the importance of chromium in nutrition. A study giving 4 micromoles of chromium picolinate to patients with elevated cholesterol levels found that after six weeks the average total cholesterol level was down by 6.9 per cent.[15]

Chromium supplementation may help to improve insulin-resistant diabetics. An Israeli study showed that 200 micrograms of chromium picolinate taken daily improved insulin resistance in 62 per cent of women and 50 per cent of men with Type II diabetes.[16]

DHEA is a hormone that drops dramatically with age. Reduced levels of DHEA increase the likelihood of memory loss, muscle fatigue, bone fragility and reduced immunity. In a test of postmenopausal women taking 200 micrograms of chromium daily, their DHEA levels dropped by 10 per cent when they stopped taking it for a four-month period.[17]

Alarmingly, it is virtually impossible to get enough chromium from food — we need to eat 3000 to 4000 calories per day to get even 50 micrograms, yet the daily required amount is 200 micrograms. It appears that chromium is not well absorbed from food, but foods high in chromium are brewers yeast, broccoli, barley, whole grains, mushrooms, and liver. It is safest to limit daily supplementation to 200 micrograms and get your doctor's advice — especially if you are diabetic, as taking chromium could alter insulin requirements.

SELENIUM

Selenium is a powerful antioxidant and an essential trace mineral with diverse health-giving properties. Selenium is known to be largely missing from New Zealand soil. Selenium levels lower with age, leaving us with lowered immunity to infections, cancer, and heart disease.

There is not a lot of research available on the effects of low selenium levels on New Zealanders. Blood levels of selenium in New Zealanders have been found to be closer to normal in recent years, most probably because of the importation of wheat from selenium-rich soils in Australia and the use of this in commercial bread and cake baking. However, whether this is sufficient to meet bodily needs or is sufficient for a possible cancer prevention effect is not known.[18]

One of the most important roles of selenium is as an essential building block for the formation of glutathione peroxidase, one of the body's most critical enzymes that neutralises free radicals.

A group of researchers from several universities in the US report that selenium supplementation helped prevent cancer. The Nutritional Prevention of Cancer study group found that cancer deaths were cut in half in a group of 1312 patients who supplemented with selenium. The reduction was particularly impressive in the case of cancers of the prostate, lung, colon and rectum. The researchers were so impressed with the results of the trial that they decided to stop it early so that patients in the placebo control group could enjoy the benefits as well. They believe that selenium combats cancer by inhibiting the late-stage promotion and progression of tumours. No toxic effects of selenium were observed.[19, 20] A very recent study reports that men who supplemented with 200 micrograms of selenium per day had a three times lower risk of developing prostate cancer than the men in the placebo group.[21]

In China, researchers in the Jiansu Province have found that supplementation with 200 micrograms of selenium per day significantly lowers the risk of developing liver cancer in a high-risk population.[22]

Low levels of selenium in the blood could also make heart disease more likely. Researchers have found that selenium strengthens the body's natural antioxidant defence systems against HIV infection.[23]

Those people whose diet is low in or excludes meat, poultry, fish and eggs and emphasises vegetables, fruit and unrefined foods — particularly those grown in a selenium-deficient soil as they are in New Zealand — may well be lacking essential selenium. A Swedish study noted that zinc and copper levels were also lower in vegetarians but that there was a significant reduction in lead, mercury and cadmium in lactovegetarians.[24]

Selenium has also been found to protect against mercury poisoning. It is believed that selenium acts by counteracting the effects of free radicals generated by the mercury. The researchers also report that deficiencies in calcium, iron and zinc enhance the toxic effects of lead by increasing the amounts of lead absorbed through the intestine.[25]

Selenium can be toxic if taken in high doses. The safe recommended daily dose is 200 micrograms per day. (To get a toxic effect you would need to eat about 2500 micrograms.) Selenium is found in grains, sunflower seeds, garlic (provided they are grown in selenium-rich soil) as well as seafood and seaweeds. A very rich source of selenium is the Brazil nut — particularly imported nuts in the shell.

CALCIUM

It has already been noted that calcium is an essential nutrient for normal growth and development and that it may lower blood pressure and cholesterol levels, prevent the development of diabetes and protect against colon and rectal cancer (see Chapters 7 and 9).

The best form of calcium supplement is calcium citrate. Dolomite and bone meal products commonly available may be high in aluminium and lead. Calcium citrate is most absorbable and is milder to take. Take in the evening for maximum absorption.

12
SECRETS OF A LONG AND HEALTHY LIFE

People say that what we're all seeking is a meaning for life. I don't think that's what we are really seeking. I think that what we're seeking is an experience of being alive, so that our life experiences on the purely physical plane will have resonances within our innermost being and reality, so that we actually feel the rapture of being alive.

Joseph Campbell

The mid-life woman is poised to move into a life phase that is liberated from the constraints of child-rearing and the effects of hormonal fluctuations. It is a time when huge personal development can take place and new life experiences can bring rich rewards. Mid-life is a time that calls for a reassessment of priorities, and may require significant lifestyle adjustments to assure us a long healthy life in which to enjoy the abundant possibilities on offer. Not only must our personal reality be addressed, the environmental issues that profoundly affect our future can no longer be ignored either.

TREAT YOURSELF! — EAT WELL

At mid-life we enter one of the most nutritionally challenging times of our life. At menopause our need for nutrients increases, while our slower metabolism means our need for calories decreases. In addition there is growing evidence that our bodies follow a genetically controlled programme that gradually reduces our defence against free radicals. This includes a reduction in our ability to absorb antioxidants (free-radical scavengers) from our diet along with other essential vitamins and minerals. We must compensate by increasing our intake of antioxidant- and nutrient-rich foods.

Fortunately all the current research and dietary suggestions for general good health, an easy menopause, and avoiding osteoporosis, heart disease, and breast cancer say the same thing: eat antioxidant-, mineral-, vitamin-, fibre- and plant hormone-rich foods. In other words, lots of fresh leafy greens and other vegetables, plenty of fruit, nuts, seeds and whole grains. The current recommendation is that we should eat at least five servings of fruit and vegetables per day, but researchers are beginning to say that the optimum intake for free-radical neutralisation is more like 12 servings a day.

A rich source of vitamins, minerals and protein are sea vegetables or seaweeds, which contain high amounts of calcium, phosphorus, selenium, magnesium, boron, iron, iodine and sodium. What we have to limit is fat, sugar, caffeine, soft drinks, heavy meat and alcohol. It is wise to supplement with essential minerals and at the very least the antioxidant vitamins C and E, and other powerful antioxidant supplements like Amrit Kalash. We must eat organically grown food, and avoid additives, preservatives, hydrogenated fats in products like margarine, and chemical sweeteners. As a precaution, steer clear of foods that may be genetically engineered and, as a consumer, demand your rights for labelling of these products.

You may like to consider the evidence that vegetarians live longer! A recent 10-year German study of 1900 vegetarians found that their mortality rate was only half that of the German population as a whole. The death rate from cardiovascular disease for male vegetarians was only 39 per cent of that of the general population and overall cancer deaths were only 48 per cent. Among female vegetarians the death rate from endocrine (hormone-related) diseases was only 19 per cent of that of the general population and the death rate from cardiovascular disease was 46 per cent. Vegetarians who exercised had half the risk of dying of heart disease than those who didn't exercise, and vegetarians of more than 20 years had half the risk of dying from cancer than those who had been vegetarians for less than 20 years.[1]

AVOID EXPOSURE TO ENVIRONMENTAL AND DOMESTIC CHEMICALS

As we prepare for the arrival of the new millennium we must deal with a continuing explosion of free radicals in the environment. We are ingesting them in ever-increasing quantities as a result of chemicals on and in our food, electromagnetic radiation, motor vehicle emissions, cigarette smoke, and stress. Our bodies are under constant assault from free radicals, which damage our cells and are believed to be at the basis of virtually all diseases and premature ageing. Some of this damage can be averted through lifestyle changes and the powerful neutralising effects of naturally occurring antioxidants. Survival into the third millennium and the survival of our children and their children requires measures to adapt to the hazards of life in these times. Having addressed our own needs, and become conscious of the critical state of the environment, we may find ourselves in a position to take action to ensure that future generations have a world to live in.

We are exposed daily to environmental and chemical dangers — many that we do not realise are in our everyday household products. For example, if you use certain household cleaners, shampoo, sunscreen, body lotions, make-up or hair dyes, you are quite possibly exposing yourself to carcinogenic by-products, or substances that react to form potent carcinogens during storage or use. While products may be labelled to tell us whether they are caustic or flammable, food and other products are not labelled with known carcinogenic ingredients and contaminants. The incidence of cancer in industrialised countries has increased by 50 per cent since 1980. This equates to one person in ten in 1950 and now one person in three in 1997. Genetics has nothing to do with this. It is the result of avoidable exposures to carcinogens in consumer products, in the air, in water or the workplace.[2] Where possible avoid using chemicals in the home, and purchase household cleaners, cosmetics and bathroom products that are guaranteed carcinogen free.

Lake Rotorua is now reputed to be as polluted as the Rhine, and a recent report from the Ministry for the Environment reveals that Auckland has higher levels of toxic organochlorine chemicals like deadly dioxin, PCBs and DDT in its air, water and soil than other parts of the country.[3] Organochlorines are caused by motor vehicle emissions, industrial processes and wastes, and pesticides and herbicides in waterways and urban soils. Tampons, sanitary pads, and toilet papers that have been bleached contain organochlorines. They are the chemicals that can cause rampant free-radical damage and hormone dysfunction resulting in cancer, allergies, hypersensitivity, nervous system damage, reproductive disorders, immune system and hormonal system disruption. Avoiding these hazards is obviously more difficult, but knowing the danger can help us make safer lifestyle decisions, and our joint concerns may prompt greater public resistance to the unchecked use of chemicals in this country.

DISCOVER WHAT BRINGS YOU JOY AND DO THAT

Doing what you love to do in life will bring you happiness, motivation, and most probably success. It will also make you energetic and highly resistant to ageing and disease. Discovering what it is that you most enjoy, and doing that, is one of the most powerful techniques for a long and healthy life. Stop somebody in the street and ask them two questions — are you happy and do you enjoy your work? If they can say yes to both questions, the chances are that they will be well. Modern medical advancement is beginning to acknowledge the effect of the mind on the body and vice versa, but is still in its infancy in terms of applying this crucial understanding to its methods of treatment.

Mind–body medicine acknowledges that our mind and body operate inseparably. For example, watching a regular diet of funny movies has been shown to cure life-threatening disease. Norman Cousins, a leader in America's intellectual community, in 1964 developed the severe condition of ankylosing spondylitis. He had a tremendous will to live and set himself the task of mobilising all the natural resources of his body and mind to combat the disease. He rejected conventional treatment and instead forged ahead with a self-prescribed regimen built on high doses of both vitamin C and laughter. He enjoyed a steady diet of *Candid Camera* and the Marx Brothers and found that 'ten minutes of genuine belly laughter had an anesthetic effect and would give me at least two hours of painfree sleep'. Cousins recovered and more than 10 years later wrote a landmark article in the *New England Journal of Medicine* and a book called *Anatomy of an Illness*.[4] His breakthrough generated an unprecedented interest in mind–body medicine.

In another example of the mind–body connection, it has been observed and verified that sudden deep shock or grief can bring on menopause. In a 15-year follow-up of breast cancer patients, researchers concluded that a woman's attitude affected whether or not the cancer spread. Those women who felt hopeless, passive and fearful had a poor outcome while those with a 'fighting spirit' appeared to live longer.[5]

Studies have shown that more people die of heart attacks on a Monday morning at 9 am than on any other day of the week. Researchers at the University of Berlin studied 5500 cases of heart attack and sudden cardiac death over five years. They found that among people who went to work, the risk of having a heart attack was 33 per cent higher on a Monday than on any other day of the week. They concluded that this was a result of a rise in blood pressure and body temperature due to an increase in physical and mental stress.[6]

A recent Harvard School of Public Health study showed that men who were inclined to worry, particularly about social conditions, the nation's economy and so on, have a 50 per cent greater chance of developing heart disease.[7] And adults who have had a troubled childhood are far more likely to have a poor health status and suffer from heart disease, diabetes, emphysema, and other common diseases.[8, 9]

EXERCISE

Maintaining a level of fitness from 40 years on is an investment in health, *joie de vivre*, energy and strength. It is possible to get away with a minimum of exercise when we are younger, but for a multitude of reasons it becomes essential once we reach mid-life. We know this, yet for many of us exercising is all too easy to avoid through lack of time and energy. In reality, though, it repays us with more time, more energy, and a renewed sense of well-being. Once a part of your routine, exercise becomes essential. It is relaxing, a mood-enhancer, will help you sleep, keep weight at normal levels and at menopause will help keep hot flushes at bay.

Regular exercise will also protect against:
- Stroke[10]
- Osteoporosis
- Heart disease
- Diabetes
- Depression
- Breast cancer[11]

Living in the nineties works against us being physically active. In fact, it continues to get easier to avoid exercising. Daily activity is geared towards working our bodies less and less as technology replaces physical effort. We no longer wrestle with the mangle to wring the clothes, mow the lawns with a push-mower, or walk to the shops and carry home the groceries as many of our mother's generation did. Many of us sit for hours in front of computer terminals and now send much of our mail electronically — threatening even to deny us the walk to the letterbox! Power steering in the car leaves arm muscles unexercised . . . escalators and lifts waft us from floor to floor and, when we shop, car parks often adjoin malls and shopping centres for ease of entry.

No group is at higher risk for depression, disease and early death than people who are completely sedentary. Studies from the Russian space programme showed that young cosmonauts subjected to the forced inactivity of space flight fell prey to depression. When they were put on a schedule of regular exercise, however, the depression was avoided.[12]

Physiologists used to believe that exercise primarily benefits us at young ages when muscles are in their prime developmental stage. However, research with the elderly has conclusively demonstrated that a person can take up exercise at any age — even centenarians will receive the same increase in strength, stamina, and muscle mass as a younger person.[13] A very new study indicates that regular exercise may also reduce the risk of developing Alzheimer's disease. The study examined the long-term health habits of 373 people — 126 of them with Alzheimer's disease and 247 of them healthy. The patients with Alzheimer's disease had had lower levels of physical activity earlier in life.[14]

But despite our knowledge of these things (and the message on the importance of exercise cannot have escaped us by now), many women still find exercising a problem. Studies have shown that women exercise less than men, and older women least of all.

In her book *Feeling Fabulous at 40, 50 and Beyond*, Sandra Coney comments on the Life in New Zealand (LINZ) survey conducted by the Hillary Commission in 1990 which revealed that among women over 50 years of age only 12 per cent took part in organised sport and 9 per cent took part in informal sport — a total of 21 per cent. 'When women stopped leisure activities, the main reason they gave for doing so were physical inability to do it, family and work commitments, lack of time, and lack of energy. These reasons identify barriers to women taking up exercise, but there are many more reasons than this. Even when they do have the time, women avoid physical activity. Women have mental barriers to taking up exercise. These relate to things such as lack of confidence, physical incompetence, lack of knowledge about sport, fear of risk-taking, embarrassment, and a dislike of competition.'[15]

It is vital that exercise gives more energy than it takes — a consideration that some people tend to ignore. Exercise should enjoyably prepare you for work, not be the work itself. The key to enjoyable exercise is not to strain. Find ways to exercise while doing something you love. Gardening is excellent and walking one of the easiest and best. A brisk half-hour walk every day will stimulate digestion, eliminate impurities in the system, clear the mind, tone the muscles, and give you a more positive perspective on life. Not surprisingly, studies show that walkers live longer. Researchers from nine American universities and health institutions conclude that regular walking increases longevity and that the risk of death can be reduced by 19 per cent for every one mile increase in daily walking distance.[16]

Dancing can be a particularly exhilarating and delightful way to exercise. Usually the pleasure of the experience overrides the sense that you are even exercising. Jude has taken up Ceroc dancing lately and believes that we don't move or dance enough in our culture. 'When we dance, the mind, body and spirit are all engaged at once. Ceroc is great fun, very sociable and quite addictive. When you move from person to person as you do with this form of dance, it mixes up the ages — cuts right through ageism. It's energising, blissful and a wonderful form of exercise.

'When I was doing relief work in Africa, I would sometimes see women singing and running together across the plains in that unique rhythmical dance-like way that they do. And I was so inspired by these people who had no possessions, lived hand-to-mouth in war zones, but still loved to dance. They would start playing the tom toms in the evening and dance all night. There was such a sense of energy and joy created.'

From an Ayur-Vedic perspective, it is best to exercise to 50 per cent of your capacity. For example, if you feel you can extend yourself to bike six miles, then do three. If you can swim 40 laps, make it 20. The point of this is that exercising to your lower limits makes exercise more efficient because your cardiovascular system will have an easier time returning to normal, and your body doesn't have to repair any damage done. It is not a good idea to over-exert. A general rule is to exercise until you break out in a light sweat only — not a heavy sweat — and just until you begin to breathe through your mouth rather than your nose. These are natural signals that you are at the right limit.

As you continue to exercise you will find that you are able to exercise for longer before the body signals that you have reached your limit.

A balanced approach to exercise is to include yoga in your daily routine. The sun salute (suryanamaskar) in particular is an excellent morning exercise that combines stretching, balance and aerobic exercise. It is a complete Ayur-Vedic exercise that simultaneously integrates the whole physiology — mind, body and breath. It strengthens and stretches all the major muscle groups, lubricates the joints, conditions the spine, stimulates blood flow and circulation and massages the internal organs! (See sun salute diagram on pages 222–223)

MEDITATION OR RELAXATION

Stress is created by an overload of experience and is acknowledged as the leading cause of disease and death in developed countries. It is not the actual situations themselves that are to blame, but rather our inability to cope with stressful situations and stimuli. Stress is generated by the tensions and pressures of work and home life, and the constant shortage of time most people live with. We face traffic stress, daily doses of stressful news broadcasts, ever-present crime. All of this stress is metabolised by the body. We have developed a society that makes us sick!

According to Dr Hari Sharma in his book *Freedom From*

Disease, 'Chronic stress leads to mental frustration, anxiety and ultimately depression. Chronic stress also breaks out physically as headaches, allergies, ulcers, and heart disease. Ultimately stress wears the immune system down and the body comes prey to disease. Sooner or later, chronic untreated stress will make you ill.'[17]

Regular daily practice of meditation is well known to reduce stress levels, and improve health and well-being. Undoubtedly the most fundamental and essential element of our daily routine, it allows the body to repair damage from the effects of stress and emotional overload, reduces fatigue and cultivates a balanced approach to life. Over the past two decades researchers have thoroughly investigated this topic and have concluded that despite appearances, not all relaxation techniques are the same. Hailed as the most extensively researched form of meditation, Transcendental Meditation (TM), with over 500 studies published in 35 years on its wide-ranging benefits, repeatedly stands out as the most effective and simple technique to reduce stress and give profoundly deep rest to the mind and body.

In a large exhaustive study published in the *Journal of Clinical Psychology*, nearly two decades of stress-related studies and various meditation and relaxation techniques were compared statistically. In the results of all the tests together, TM was shown to reduce anxiety twice as much as any other technique.[18]

TM has also been shown to:
- reduce depression and aggression
- normalise blood pressure comparably with conventional drug treatment
- reduce biological ageing
- help prevent cancer and heart disease
- reduce hospital admissions by 50 per cent overall

A massive study measuring 2000 people practising TM over a five-year period and comparing them to other groups of similar age, gender, profession and insurance terms found that the TM group had 87 per cent less hospitalisation for heart disease, 55 per cent less for cancer, 87 per cent less for nervous system disorders and 73 per cent less for nose, throat and lung problems.[19]

More than releasing stress and reducing the risk of disease, meditation, and again in particular TM because of its simplicity and effortlessness, brings the value of that innermost field of silence, creativity, energy and bliss into our awareness. The sense of being connected with one's self, at home in that most settled state of awareness, naturally results in increased naturalness, peaceful rewarding relationships, and a sense that all is in order in one's life.

SUMMARY OF STRATEGIES FOR A LONG FULFILLING LIFE

1. Practice meditation or relaxation daily.
2. Eat a nutrient-rich diet full of natural organic fresh foods — avoid genetically modified organisms. Avoid saturated and polyunsaturated fats — favour monounsaturated fats.
3. Eat antioxidant-rich foods and supplements. Supplement with essential minerals and vitamins.
4. Do what you love to do — it makes you highly resistant to disease and the negative effects of ageing.
5. Exercise!
6. Avoid smoking and alcohol.
7. Try to have less exposure to chemical pollution.

The perils of modern life are many, but so are the solutions. By living wisely and applying simple strategies such as those outlined in this book, we can expect to comfortably negotiate menopause and continue to grow and develop as individuals. Provided we achieve a balance of healthy mind and body, mid-life marks the passage to our new role as wise, liberated women in our communities.

Above all, we must look for happiness in whatever we pursue.

The purpose of life is the expansion of happiness. Mid-life for women is a transition that demands change. It offers a wonderful opportunity to reassess our lifestyle, be re-educated, and adopt new strategies to launch ourselves into what can be the most fulfilling and productive phase of our lives.

As enlightened women in our communities we can use our influence and life experience to demand a safer environment for our children and grandchildren, and to ask the questions that need to be asked of the policy-makers. The new millennium demands change also.

13
NATURAL SOLUTIONS FOR COMMON SYMPTOMS OF MENOPAUSE

There are many simple, effective ways to address the symptoms of menopause, the simplest of all being to eat well, exercise regularly and nourish both mind and body with good routine, deep rest and relaxation. This should help you avoid any difficulties. However, if you do experience specific uncomfortable symptoms, the following suggestions may be helpful. Some methods work brilliantly for some, and not so well for others. We are all different, and it is impossible to predict which herb or therapy will work best for you. Often it is a case of trial and error, so for this reason it is probably a good idea to try only one option at a time.

The following dietary herbal and other suggestions are summaries from the information given throughout the book. The majority of these suggestions are traditional nutritional remedies, which are side-effect and risk free. There will always be a small percentage of people who have allergic or other reactions to even the mildest of herbs, and for this reason we emphasise the need to go by the stated dose, and recommend that you begin with the lowest dose, and take it throughout the day in divided doses.

Although most of the treatment options that follow are well researched and have stood the test of time and experience, some have not yet been subjected to scientific scrutiny in well-designed trials.

HOT FLUSHES AND NIGHT SWEATS

Up to 80 per cent of women have hot flushes at menopause, but only in about 10 per cent of women are they severe. They do eventually stop, often within a year or two. Fortunately there are some effective ways to reduce or eliminate them.

NUTRITION

Include more of the foods that are high in hormonally active compounds (phytoestrogens) in your diet.

Excellent sources of phytoestrogens are:
- Legumes: soybeans, lentils, beans (haricot, broad, kidney, lima), chickpeas, sprouted soy and alfalfa
- Soybean products: soy milk, soy flour, soy grits, tofu, tempeh (make sure soy products are organic)
- Whole-grain cereals: wheat, wheatgerm, barley, hops, rye, rice, bran, oats
- Fruit, vegetables and seeds: cherries, apples, pears, stone fruits, celery, fennel, green and yellow vegetables (including kumara), anise and licorice, rhubarb and linseed (flaxseed), olive oil

Vegetable proteins are much easier for your body to digest and use than animal proteins. Good sources are: legumes, grains, nuts and seeds (whole and sprouted).

Avoid foods that trigger hot flushes like caffeine, alcohol and spicy foods.

TRY TAKING A SUPPLEMENT

Health-food stores offer an array of herbs and supplements in

NATURAL SOLUTIONS

various combinations. Most of them are phytoestrogen- and micronutrient-rich traditional treatments and are well worth trying. Remember to try only one supplement at a time (so that you know what works) and always go by the stated dose. It may be a good idea to discuss the best regime for you with your health practitioner.

- Vitamin E 400 IU and selenium (150 mcg) work together. Take with meals containing oils or fats.
- Ginseng is also a type of phytoestrogen known as a saponin and has been used for thousands of years in Asia for reproductive disorders. Some women find that sipping ginseng tea is helpful.
- Evening primrose oil
- Herbal remedies, for example, black cohosh, sage, red clover, chaste tree, motherwort, false unicorn
- $1/2$ cup sage tea at bedtime for night sweats
- Natural progesterone
- Bee pollen products
- Soy products

EXERCISE

Hot flushes can be significantly reduced by exercising as little as 20 minutes three times a week. Walking is great, so is swimming, cycling, dancing, tramping, playing tennis, etc.

ACUPUNCTURE

Acupuncture can be very effective in relieving hot flushes. It usually requires one or two treatments only and repeat treatments when and if symptoms return.

Ayur-Vedic treatments like panchakarma, herbs and daily routine can successfully eliminate the uncomfortable symptoms of menopause.

INSOMNIA

The diet and lifestyle recommendations listed above could be helpful for insomnia. You could also try:

- Herbal remedies: valerian, passion flower, St John's wort, chamomile tea, hops. Sage tea (1/2 cup) before bed calms and helps sleep.
- Natural progesterone is reported by many women to bring excellent results.
- Warm milk helps induce sleepiness and calcium taken at night is better absorbed and helps you to sleep.
- Meditation/relaxation techniques practised regularly will usually eliminate insomnia.
- Eating lightly in the evening — an important principle of Ayur-Veda — but don't go to bed really hungry either.
- Magnesium supplementation of 200mg daily.
- Decrease caffeine and alcohol, especially at night.
- Exercise daily.
- Aromatherapy — a few drops of essential oil in the bath or in an oil diffuser can be soothing and aid sleep. Try the menopause oils geranium, lavender, or bergamot.
- Ayur-Vedic treatments — see a practitioner.

ANXIETY/DEPRESSION (MILD)

Some women experience mood swings and unexplained episodes of sadness at menopause. Mood swings may in part be due to lack of sleep, but may also be helped by the following:

- St John's wort, kava kava (see Chapter 10).
- Vitamin B_6 and magnesium.
- The herb black cohosh, typically prescribed for hot flushes, is also calming, and has been shown to be helpful for mood swings, anxiety and depression when combined with St John's wort.[1]
- Reducing alcohol.

- Exercising regularly.
- Taking time out for you — it is very important to find at least an hour or two every day to make your own needs a priority.
- Meditation or relaxation. Studies have shown that TM reduces anxiety twice as effectively as all other forms of relaxation or meditation.[2]

VAGINAL DRYNESS

Reduced levels of female hormones at mid-life cause the tissues of the vagina to become thinner, dryer and more prone to infection. Normal vaginal secretions decline and intercourse can be painful. There are a number of successful treatments available.

- Herbs: Chaste tree or vitex taken orally as a herb or wild yam vaginal gel.
- Vitamin E oil-based capsule — 100 IU inserted in the vagina every night for six weeks will help restore tissue and mucosa.
- A tampon soaked in very fine linseed or sesame oil and inserted in the vagina daily for two to three hours can be restorative, healing and soothing.
- Natural progesterone cream is reported to be effective.
- Oestrogen creams prescribed by your doctor can be very helpful. Be aware, however, that although providing a lower level of oestrogen it is a still a form of HRT.
- Calendula, aloe vera, comfrey, or turmeric creams applied externally are soothing for dryness and itchiness.
- Regular sexual intercourse will help preserve vaginal tissue, perhaps by increasing blood flow to the area.
- There are several excellent water-based lubricants available at your pharmacy including Astroglyde, and Sylke — a kiwifruit-derived New Zealand-made product. (Avoid if you are allergic to kiwifruit though!) Don't use petroleum-based lubricants as they may cause irritation.

LOSS OF SEX DRIVE OR LIBIDO

Many women find they experience less interest in sex at mid-life, which can have distressing consequences for them. Libido is often a general indicator of health, and likely to be affected if you are not sleeping well, and are experiencing hot flushes, mood swings and irritability. But it is also related to the changing balance of hormones in your body and will often be helped by increasing your intake of phytoestrogens and particularly the herbs known to increase libido. Many women report that natural progesterone cream has restored their sex drive to premenopausal levels. Some women benefit from small amounts of the hormone testosterone, now available on prescription in a nature-identical cream form. It is vital that you talk to your partner and develop an understanding; maybe explore other ways of expressing sexuality.

The recommended herbs are: chaste tree (see Chapter 5), wild yam or damiana.

STRESS INCONTINENCE/ URINARY PROBLEMS

Lower levels of hormones can cause the tissues lining the bladder to become thinner, making it easier for bladder infections (urinary-tract infections) to develop. To prevent infections, try the following:

- Drink lots of water — particularly warm or hot water. This will keep the bladder full and flushing frequently, so the level of bacteria in the bladder is diluted. Avoid caffeine and alcohol as, being diuretics, they are more likely to encourage dehydration.
- Urinate frequently, especially after sex, as this will prevent bacterial concentration.
- Do your pelvic floor exercises — at least 100 times every day! They help to keep muscles strong and reduce urinary frequency and likelihood of infection. Do them while you are waiting at the lights, or in the supermarket queue. Try putting coloured dots around the house — in the bathroom or above the sink — to remind you!

- Take cranberry as a dried fruit or juice (unsweetened) or in capsule form. Cranberry is a bioflavanoid and has an active ingredient that is believed to prevent bacteria from clinging to the wall of the urinary tract where they can multiply and cause infection and painful urination. A six-month study of postmenopausal elderly women showed that drinking 10 ounces of cranberry juice a day lowered the amount of bacteria and white blood cells in the urine.[3]

ACHING JOINTS

Often mistaken for arthritis, joints, legs, and feet can develop inexplicable aches and pains at menopause, which come and go. Treatments to try are:

- St John's wort, which has anti-inflammatory properties, and evening primrose oil, which is well known as a successful treatment for joint pain and rheumatoid arthritis.
- Calcium/magnesium/potassium supplements, as joint pain can be due to a mineral deficiency.
- A small amount (a quarter of a teaspoon) of natural progesterone cream rubbed onto the site of pain.
- Massage to soothe and ease pain.

MEMORY LOSS

A gradual loss of memory performance is often part of the ageing process, and many researchers believe that the process is intimately associated with free-radical damage. Antioxidants are once again a priority. Supplementing with vitamins C and E has been found to be helpful. A recent study at the University of Berne showed that among participants aged 65 years or older a high level of vitamin C and beta-carotene is closely related to better memory performance. The researchers concluded that antioxidants play an important role in the prevention of memory loss related to brain ageing.[4]

A deficiency of the essential fatty acids in our diet (found in fresh vegetables, nuts, seeds and whole grains), coupled with too much saturated fat (for example, butter and animal fat) can affect levels of the hormone prolactin, a hormone that appears to be particularly bound up with premenstrual and menopausal symptoms. Supplementation with gamma-linolenic acid in the form of evening primrose oil has been reported to help memory loss associated with menopause.

Gingko biloba has a long history of use in treating mental problems and is currently used widely in Europe. It is recommended for short-term memory loss, slowed reaction time, low energy levels, and difficulty concentrating and staying alert. Its main benefit is the increase of blood circulation, which researchers suggest may lessen many of the complaints that come about as a result of insufficient arterial blood supply to the brain.

ALZHEIMER'S DISEASE

Although Alzheimer's disease is not associated with menopause, it is an age-related condition that is afflicting more and more people. Clinical studies with *Gingko biloba* have shown promising results in the areas of memory loss, senile dementia, Alzheimer's disease, and other age-related diseases. Most recently, a team of medical doctors including researchers from the Harvard Medical School, the Albert Einstein College of Medicine, and the New York Medical College report that *Ginkgo biloba* extract is effective in slowing down and, in some cases, reversing the progression of Alzheimer's disease. The effect was most pronounced on the subjects who were the least impaired, suggesting that if Alzheimer's is treated early enough, dementia might be postponed.[5]

There is growing evidence that severe memory loss and Alzheimer's disease involves oxidative stress and an accumulation of free radicals which leads to neuronal degeneration in the brain. Now researchers at Columbia University report that vitamin E, a powerful lipid-soluble antioxidant, is very effective in slowing the progression of Alzheimer's disease.[6]

Another new study indicates that regular exercise may reduce the risk of developing Alzheimer's disease. The study examined the long-term health habits of 373 people — 126 with Alzheimer's disease and 247 healthy. The patients with Alzheimer's disease had lower levels of physical activity earlier in life.[7]

Note: Anyone experiencing memory lapses should first consult a physician.

HEADACHES

Changes in hormone levels can trigger headaches in some women. Fortunately they tend to diminish and disappear after menopause. Many headaches, including migraine, are triggered by certain foods, which once identified can be avoided.

Common trigger foods are:
- Alcohol — particularly red wine and beer
- Tyramine in aged cheeses, chianti wine and some pickled herring
- Chocolate

HELPFUL TREATMENTS:
- Feverfew, St John's wort, chaste tree
- Vitamin B_2
- Evening primrose oil, effective in the treatment of migraine[8]
- Magnesium (220mg) daily in a chelated form can help reduce headaches. The body's requirement for magnesium increases at mid-life
- Fresh ginger tea taken at the onset of a headache can prevent it setting in
- Avoid tea and coffee
- Natural progesterone can be very effective for hormone-related headache as it counteracts the dilation of vessels that causes the headache[9]
- Meditation and relaxation techniques
- Yoga

SKIN PROBLEMS

Dryness, itchiness, and skin changes may be helped by taking the herbs echinacea, chaste tree or burdock. Skin problems could be related to a deficiency in essential fatty acids. Supplementing with evening primrose oil may therefore be helpful. Turmeric cream has remarkable anti-inflammatory and healing properties and is excellent for most skin conditions.

MENSTRUAL FLOODING

- Herbs: Ginseng, sage, chaste tree. These herbs help to restore hormonal balance as they contain phytohormones. Always buy the best (therefore purest) ginseng you can afford. Take either as a fresh root tincture or as a tea in which 24 g of dried root or paste is taken in hot water (avoid the Chinese herb dong quai).
- Acupuncture can be very effective.
- Natural progesterone can help regulate your cycle and reduce bleeding.

FATIGUE

It is a good idea to get your iron and mineral levels checked. Regular exercise can usually restore energy levels. But listen to your body too and if you are tired, rest more, and look at your diet and lifestyle. Deep rest from meditation can be more effective than napping and can help to release stress and restore your energy reserves.

WEIGHT GAIN

Apply the Ayur-Vedic principles and eat only when you are hungry. Drink warm or hot water throughout the day. Reduce intake of saturated and processed polyunsaturated fats. Avoid sugar, sweets, chocolate and other foods high in calories and low in nutritional value. Eat lots of low-calorie, low-fat, high-fibre, antioxidant-rich nutritious food: fresh fruit, vegetables, whole grains and seeds.

Limit or avoid alcohol and coffee. Exercise regularly. Many women have had great results with the Liver Cleansing Diet, which applies the above recommendations.[10]

FLUID RETENTION

- Herbs: juniper, parsley, or watermelon seeds
- Evening primrose oil

BREAST TENDERNESS

It is common to feel breast pain or breast tenderness at menopause. Some women have more breast pain when they are under stress. Natural progesterone has been reported to be very helpful.

Some women with breast pain have been shown to have low levels of gamma-linolenic acid, and treatment with evening primrose oil has brought relief.

RECIPES

Fresh organic vegetables, fruit, sea vegetables, nuts, seeds and legumes provide us with antioxidants, minerals, vitamins and plant hormones. Wonderful recipes abound for these foods, so we offer only a small selection here. These are samples of mainly Asian-style recipes along with some basic Ayur-Vedic recipes. Asian and Indian food stores can supply the ingredients.

PHYTOESTROGENS

Some of the following recipes include soy products like tofu which provide an excellent source of plant hormone. It is important to remember that the soy bean is now genetically engineered. At this time you can still avoid genetically engineered soy and other foods by eating organic products. Soy is only one of many plants that are high in plant hormone — there are plenty of alternatives.

Japanese Asparagus Soba Noodles

This dish is simple and quick to make, provides delicious clean light flavours and is very nutritious.

250g pack soba (buckwheat) noodles
6–8 cups water
250g packet tempeh
Soy sauce or tamari
2 tablespoons olive oil
1/4 cup dried hijiki (sea vegetable)
2 teaspoons peeled fresh ginger, grated
2 bunches asparagus, cut into 2cm pieces
1 carrot cut into thin strips
2 courgettes cut into strips
200g snow-pea shoots

Cook the noodles according to package instructions. Refresh under cold running water, drain well, and set aside. Slice tempeh into small pieces and brush with tamari. Sauté in skillet with olive oil until lightly browned. Soak the hijiki in 1 cup of boiling water for 10 minutes until it swells. Drain. Sauté the grated ginger in heated olive oil for 10 seconds. Add the asparagus, carrot and courgettes. Stir fry until vegetables are tender. Add snow-pea shoots. Combine all ingredients, add a little tamari to taste and serve immediately. Serves 4.

Thai-style Tofu Curry

This favourite is quick to prepare, nutritious and very satisfying.

250g organic tofu
2 tablespoons olive oil
1/2 teaspoon Thai green curry paste
1 400ml can coconut milk
2 teaspoons peeled fresh ginger, chopped
2 small red capsicums, seeded and sliced

200g snow-pea shoots
1 bunch spinach, washed and cut into pieces
2 courgettes, cut into strips
1 bunch asparagus (optional), cut into pieces
2 tablespoons fresh coriander
2 tablespoons fresh lemon juice

Sauté tofu in a little olive oil. When lightly browned add green curry paste. Sauté for about 10 seconds then add coconut milk. Heat and leave. In a separate skillet sauté ginger in heated olive oil for 10 seconds. Add prepared vegetables and stir-fry until tender. Add chopped coriander and lemon juice to vegetables. Combine all and serve over jasmine or basmati rice. Serves 4.

Organic Tofu Dressing

Serve over a hearty, crunchy salad of slivered carrots, celery, red pepper, chopped bok choy and chunks of tofu. Also try with a fruit salad of papaya, pineapple and apples. Add more wasabi if you prefer it extra hot.

250g organic tofu
1 tablespoon rice vinegar
2 teaspoons olive oil
2 teaspoons wasabi powder
1 teaspoon minced shallot or spring onion
1 teaspoon each lemon juice, sesame oil, and soy sauce
½ teaspoon minced ginger root
4 tablespoons water
Salt and pepper to taste

In a blender, mix together all ingredients, stopping to scrape down sides as necessary, until smooth. Makes about ¾ cup.

Caesar Salad and Creamy Dressing

This version of the classic has a bold, zesty flavour and includes the nutritional boost and taste of nori (seaweed). Toss with Romaine lettuce, croutons, cheese and freshly ground black pepper.

250g organic tofu
1 tablespoon slivered blanched almonds
2 cloves garlic, minced
1 tablespoon fresh lemon juice
1 tablespoon prepared mustard
1 tablespoon extra virgin olive oil
1 tablespoon nutritional yeast
1 teaspoon soy sauce
1/2 sheet nori, torn into pieces

In a blender, mix together all ingredients, stopping to scrape down sides as necessary, until smooth. Makes about 1 cup.

Tofu Dressing with Sun-Dried Tomatoes

This thick dressing doubles beautifully as a spread over broiled tempeh. Add more liquid from the soaked tomatoes if you prefer a thinner dressing.

6 sun-dried tomato halves (not oil-packed)
1/4 cup boiling water
250g organic tofu
1 or 2 teaspoons prepared wasabi
1 tablespoon tomato paste
1 teaspoon minced chives or spring onion
1/2 teaspoon soy sauce
Salt and pepper to taste

In a small bowl, cover sun-dried tomatoes with boiling water and let sit until tomatoes have softened, 15–20 minutes. Remove tomatoes and chop coarsely; reserve soaking liquid. In a blender, combine tomatoes with remaining ingredients. Blend until smooth, stopping to scrape down sides 2 or 3 times. Add liquid, as needed, to achieve desired consistency. Makes about 1 cup.

Creamy Sesame Miso Dressing

Great with spinach and potato salads, or to dress up chilled slices of fresh tofu.

250g organic tofu
2 tablespoons light miso paste dissolved in a little warm water
2 tablespoons organic soy milk or water
1 tablespoon cider vinegar
1 teaspoon sesame oil
Pepper to taste

In a blender, mix together all ingredients, stopping to scrape down sides as necessary, until smooth. Makes about $3/4$ cup.

SEA VEGETABLES

'Sea vegetables are a delicacy fit for the most honored guest,' wrote Sze Tsu while studying with Confucius in the 6th century BC.

Sea vegetables are among the most nutrient-dense foods on the planet. They are powerhouses of minerals and protein, high in potassium, selenium, calcium, iron, iodine, and chromium, as well as vitamin K. Nori has 25 per cent more protein than milk, without the fat and calories, and other sea vegetables such as arame, wakame and hijiki are exceptionally high in calcium.

Sea vegetables are available dried and packaged in Asian markets and natural food stores. Stored in airtight containers, they will keep for up to two years. If spots of white appear, they're salt crystals coming to the surface — simply wipe them away before using. Always rinse them well (with the exception of sheet nori), throw the first salty rinse water away, then soak until the vegetables are supple.

Taste and texture vary from sweet, lush, and spicy to nutty, chewy, and briny. Once you become familiar with the unique qualities of each type, you'll soon want to start experimenting. Sea vegetables invite you to cook beautiful dishes full of complex flavour and nutrition. Add a little sea life to stews and soups, stir-fries, salads, and even sandwiches.

Sushi Nori Rolls

Making sushi is easier than you might think.

1½ cups medium grain white rice
2 cups cold water
3 tablespoons seasoned rice vinegar
6 sheets roasted nori
½ cucumber, peeled, seeded and cut into 6mm strips
1 carrot, peeled, cut into 6mm strips
1 bell pepper, cut into 6mm strips
Wasabi, pickled ginger, and soy sauce (optional)

In a medium saucepan with a tight-fitting lid, combine rice and water. Bring to the boil over medium-high heat, reduce temperature to low and simmer, covered, for 10 minutes, or until all the liquid is absorbed. Remove from heat and let stand, covered, for 20 minutes. Transfer to a large mixing bowl and stir in vinegar. Set aside to cool, stirring occasionally, until rice reaches room temperature.

Fill a small bowl with cool water for moistening fingers to aid in working with the sticky rice. On a bamboo sushi mat or a flat surface, lay 1 nori sheet with longer edge closest to you. Spread ¾ cup rice evenly over the nori, allowing 12mm margin on longer edges. Place 3 or 4 strips of desired vegetables at the closest edge of the rice and press lightly. Carefully roll the sushi away from yourself, using firm and even pressure. (The rolls must be fairly tight.) Repeat, assembling the remaining ingredients into rolls.

Cut each roll into 8 pieces and serve with wasabi, pickled ginger, and soy sauce, if desired. Makes 6 rolls.

Miso Soup with Arame, Ginger and Green Onions

If you're in a hurry, skip infusing the broth with shiitake and just use hot water. Add the miso at the very end and heat gently — boiling makes miso bitter. When making a soup, there's no need to soak the sea vegetable.

4 cups water
4 dried shiitake mushrooms
1 cup thinly sliced carrot
1 cup dried arame, washed
1 tablespoon finely chopped fresh ginger
5 tablespoons miso, dissolved in 1/4 cup warm water
Soy sauce to taste
4 scallions, sliced

In a medium soup pot, bring water to a boil, turn off heat, add mushrooms, and let stand for 15 minutes, or until mushrooms are soft and water is infused with flavour. Remove mushrooms, slice, and return to pot. Over medium heat, bring broth to a slow boil, add carrots, arame, and ginger, reduce heat and simmer for 10 minutes, or until carrots are tender. Add miso/water mixture and simmer for 2 minutes. Season to taste with soy sauce and sprinkle with scallions. Serves 4.

Wakame, Spinach and Tofu

Serve over rice and sprinkle with sesame seeds.

1/2 cup dried wakame
1 clove garlic, minced
1/2 cup diced firm organic tofu
2 teaspoons sesame oil
500g fresh spinach, washed and coarsely chopped
2 teaspoons ginger juice (obtained by squeezing fresh grated ginger root through a cheesecloth)
1 teaspoon miso paste dissolved in 1 tablespoon warm water

In a medium bowl, rinse wakame. Discard rinse water, cover with fresh water, soak for 15 minutes, and drain. Trim and discard any hard membranes and chop remaining wakame. In a large skillet over medium-high heat, sauté garlic and tofu in oil for 5 minutes, or until lightly browned. Add spinach, wakame, ginger juice, and miso. Cook, stirring constantly, until spinach is just wilted, about 5 minutes. Serves 4.

Hijiki Rainbow Salad

The taste of fresh sweetcorn and tomatoes combined with salty hijiki is a summer treat.

1/2 cup dried hijiki
1 cup cherry tomatoes, halved
1 cup fresh corn kernels
1 spring onion, chopped
1 cup fresh whole or cooked peas
1/2 cup diced firm organic tofu
1 tablespoon olive oil
1/4 teaspoon sesame oil
3 tablespoons lemon juice
1 teaspoon mustard
Pepper to taste
1/2 cup fresh borage flowers (optional)

In a medium bowl, rinse hijiki. Discard rinse water, cover with fresh water, soak for 15 minutes, drain, and slice. In a large salad bowl, combine tomatoes, corn, spring onion, peas, tofu, and hijiki. In a small bowl, combine olive oil, sesame oil, lemon juice, and mustard. Dress and toss salad, and season with pepper. Garnish with borage flowers, if desired. Serves 6.

Hummus

This tasty purée is a nutritious main dish when served as a filling for whole wheat pita bread or an excellent appetiser when served with raw vegetables. It provides a good source of plant hormone and minerals from the chick-peas and tahini, a paste made from sesame seeds.

1 clove garlic
2 cups well-cooked chick-peas
Juice of 1 lemon
3–4 tablespoons cold water
¼ cup sesame tahini
½ teaspoon salt
1 tablespoon olive oil
Dash cayenne pepper, optional
Fresh coriander for garnishing

Process garlic until finely minced. Add chick-peas, lemon juice, water, tahini and salt. Process until smooth, scraping down the sides of the bowl with a spatula as needed. Taste and adjust seasoning. Spread hummus in a shallow dish. Dribble on olive oil, and garnish with cayenne pepper and coriander.

Broccoli Blue Cheese Rice
2 cups basmati rice
1½ cups small broccoli florets
½ cup diced red pepper
¼ cup sliced spring onions with tops
3 tablespoons crumbled blue cheese
3 tablespoons mayonnaise
3 tablespoons plain fresh yoghurt
1 tablespoon lemon juice
Freshly ground black pepper

Cook rice as normal, adding broccoli during the last 3 minutes of cooking. Transfer to a bowl. Cool to room temperature. Combine rice and broccoli with remaining ingredients; toss. Chill. Serve with freshly ground black pepper on a bed of mesclun salad greens. Serves 4.

AYUR-VEDA RECIPES

Important: These recipes are designed to be soothing and nourishing and to balance the three doshas, Vata, Pitta and Kapha. They are quite general and give you a glimpse of the possibilities with Ayur-Vedic cooking. They are traditional Indian vegetarian recipes which meet the Ayur-Vedic requirements.

The main meal is recommended to be in the middle of the day, cooked and hot, made of wholesome ingredients and with all six tastes included in the meal (sweet, sour, salty, bitter, pungent, astringent). It should be eaten with attention and enjoyment. Relax for 5–15 minutes after eating. It is optional, but it is actually better to eat the heaviest and richest food first — like dessert or salad, followed by the main course. You can finish with lassi or fruit.

Desserts are usually made from grains like semolina (wheat) or rice. They tend to be very sweet and rich. Only very small servings are required!

Basic Halva

1 cup semolina
125g butter
1 cup brown sugar
2 cups boiling water
$1/2$ teaspoon natural vanilla

Melt butter and add semolina. Stir over medium heat for 5 minutes then add sugar, water and vanilla stir until thick. Serves 6.

Variations: Coconut: Add $1/2$ cup of coconut with the water. Nut: Grind $1/2$ cup of almonds or hazelnuts, add to the semolina before cooking. Orange: Replace some of the water with the juice of one orange, and add the grated rind plus 1 tablespoon of golden syrup to the water before adding to the semolina (omit the vanilla). For lemon halva, add grated lemon rind.

Rice Pudding or Cereal

This recipe can also be used for sago, tapioca, barley or wheat. If it is used as a cereal for the evening meal, try it without the sugar. Serves 4–6.

1/2 cup rice (or sago, etc)
3 cups milk
1/3 cup sugar
1/2 teaspoon each of cinnamon and cardamom

Either: Mix ingredients, put in a buttered pie dish and cook in a slow oven — for rice and barley 2 hours; for sago or tapioca 1 hour (soak tapioca in milk for an hour first); for wheat 3 hours. Or: Cook in a double boiler, or stainless-steel bowl inside a large pot in about 1 litre of water. Simmer on low for about 1/2 the time for oven cooking — until grains are soft.

SALAD

Recommended are sprouts, grated carrot and beetroot, parsley, basil, freshly grated root ginger, lemon juice, black or green olives, black pepper and rock salt, churnas (seasoning mixes) to taste.

MAIN COURSE

This course alone can make up the meal. If you have a rice dish, mung dahl or other astringent food, vegetables and spices, you will have included all six tastes. You may also like to add churnas, chutneys, Indian pickles (mango, lime), roti or poppadoms.

Basmati Rice

2 cups water for every 1 cup rice

Wash rice, add water plus salt to taste, boil for 15–20 minutes. (A rice-cooker is a good investment.) **Variation**: A teaspoon each of seeds such as sunflower, sesame, mustard and poppy can be fried with a teaspoon of turmeric in 1–2 teaspoons of ghee, then stirred into the cooked rice before serving.

Mung Dahl
3 cups of water for each cup of mung dahl
Salt to taste

Simmer gently for 30 minutes, stirring occasionally. (Ghee and spices or curry powder can be added.) Allow 1/4 cup dahl per serving.

Note: A stainless-steel pressure cooker is invaluable for quick cooking of all dried beans, peas, lentils and dahl; also for cooking pearl barley in the case of Kapha imbalances and for all soups.

Spicy Vegetables
1 teaspoon (approx.) each of any of the following: turmeric, fennel, cumin, mustard seeds, caraway, ground coriander seeds
1/2 teaspoon each of cardamom and ginger (powdered or fresh grated)
1/4 teaspoon hing (asafoetida)
Black pepper and rock salt
2–3 cups diced vegetables — carrot, cauliflower, silverbeet, cabbage, spinach, etc
2 teaspoons ghee

Fry the spices you prefer in the ghee for 1–2 minutes. Stir in the vegetables. Add a little water if necessary and cook with the lid on until vegetables are just cooked (10–12 minutes). Serves 4–6.

Yoghurt can be taken with rice as part of the main meal; however, it may not be suitable for Kapha or Pitta types. It should always be eaten within 24 hours of being made. Boil the quantity of milk you want, e.g., 1 litre; let cool to 40°C (use a thermometer). Put milk into yoghurt maker or pre-heated thermos, and mix in starter — the best starter to use is powdered culture available from health shops. You can use a tablespoon of fresh yoghurt as a starter for the next batch, but commercial yoghurt will only work if it is very fresh. Check the expiry date on the container, and do not use if it is within 3–4 weeks of expiry. Leave for 5 hours or overnight. Do not refrigerate when made.

Poppadoms

These are flat discs of lentil flour and spices, available in Indian shops. They are not fresh food, but are a tasty addition to a meal and include the astringent taste. Fry for about $1/2$ minute each side in hot ghee, until lightly browned, 2 per person.

Toasted Tofu

250g firm organic tofu
$1/2$ teaspoon salt
3 tablespoons each of water, sesame seeds and flour

Dice the tofu into approx. 1cm cubes, place in bowl and sprinkle with the water. Add salt, sesame seeds and flour; either stir well or put a lid on the bowl and shake. Tip into a little hot ghee in a frying-pan and fry until crisp and light brown, stirring occasionally.

Kofta Balls

This is an easy recipe if you have a food processor to shred the vegetables. Serves 4–6.

$3^1/2$ cups finely shredded vegetables (cauliflower, broccoli, carrot, zucchini, white radish, etc)
1 cup chick-pea flour (called channa flour in Indian shops) or pea flour
$1/2$ teaspoon salt
1 tablespoon diced root ginger
1 teaspoon turmeric
1 teaspoon each of ground ginger, cumin and coriander
3 tablespoons chopped parsley
Ghee for frying

Mix all ingredients together. When the ghee is hot, form into golf-ball-sized balls by squeezing pieces of the mixture into shape, and put in hot ghee. Fry about 5 minutes each side until well browned. Serve on rice with chutney.

Roti or Chapatti

These are flat-breads which are quick and fun to make, cheap, nourishing and delicious! Allow about 1/2 cup of flour per roti and 1–2 rotis per person.

2 cups chapatti flour (bought from Indian shops) or white flour
3/4 cup warm water (approx.)

Add all the water to most of the flour, mix, then knead in more flour until the mixture stops sticking to the hands, but is still soft. Knead well, and ideally leave to sit for 30 minutes. On a floured board, cut into 4 and roll out to circles approx. 20cm diameter. Place 1 on a hot skillet or frying-pan. (Special skillets can be bought from Indian shops.) Cook until underside begins to brown, then turn over, and brush cooked side with a little butter or ghee. When roti begins to bubble, turn again, brush with butter and serve as soon as it is well cooked. Non-fat: Cook without the butter, then hold over a flame with tongs to bubble up.

Pancakes

These are delicious if you use freshly ground flour. You can substitute some of the flour with dahl flours such as channa, mung, or urid to provide the astringent taste. (You can also include whichever grain flours you prefer — rice, barley, millet, corn, oat, rye, etc.) You can prepare spicy vegetables (see recipe), and while that is cooking, mix and cook 1 or 2 pancakes — and be eating a well-balanced meal within 20 minutes of starting.

½ cup flour per pancake (approx.)
Enough water to make a runny mixture
Butter

Melt about 1 teaspoon of butter in a hot frying pan. Pour in enough mixture to cover the bottom of the pan, tipping the pan to spread the mixture. Cook until set, then turn and cook second side until browned also. Serve.

Fresh Chutney

There are many recipes for chutneys in Asian cookbooks. A basic guide is as follows:

2 cups (approx.) diced fruit (fresh, dried or a mixture) such as figs, dates, raisins, prunes, dried apricots, apples, pears, peaches, tamarillo (can include some banana)
Enough water to cook to a soft pulp (more if dried fruit is used)
1 teaspoon (approx.) each preferred spices such as cinnamon, cardamom, ground coriander, caraway seeds, cumin, turmeric
½ teaspoon cloves
Chilli powder to taste
Brown sugar to taste (approx. ½ cup)
Lemon juice and/or grated rind (optional)

Simmer all ingredients until fruit is cooked and soft. Serve hot or cold with main meal.

TO FINISH

Lassi or sweet fruit, which are easy to digest.

Lassi: Fresh-made yoghurt whipped with an equal amount of water, honey to taste and a pinch of cardamom or ginger.

THE EVENING MEAL

This meal should always be lighter than lunch, and should be eaten before 6–7 pm. Kapha types may need very little.

Soup

A very digestible soup can be made with 1/2 cup dahl, 1/2 cup basmati rice, 1 teaspoon each of cumin and chopped root ginger, and salt to taste, mixed with 4 cups of water. Can add vegetables and ghee. Simmer at least 30 minutes, or cook approx. 4 minutes in pressure-cooker — a very quick, balanced meal. Serves 2.

Fritters

Make the pancake mixture with 3 parts wheat flour to 1 part chick-pea or pea flour, slightly thicker than for pancakes. For each cup of flour used, mix in 1 1/2 mashed bananas, or 1 large apple, grated, or the kernels scraped off 1 cob of corn plus a little salt. Fry 3–4 fritters at once in a little ghee in a frying-pan. When cooked on one side, turn and cook the other side.

Roti Salad

Serve early, as salad is heavy to digest. Make roti, spread with butter, Indian pickles (mango, lime, etc) or chutneys to taste, and fill with any of the following: avocado, sprouts, tomato or cucumber slices, olives, black pepper, sliced beetroot.

A roti and a glass of lassi make a satisfying meal.

SNACKS

If you are hungry between meals, the only snacks that don't interfere with digestion are lassi and sweet fruit. If you are not sure whether you are really hungry, sip some hot water instead. (It is important to have plenty of hot water throughout the day.)

Fruit Smoothie: A substitute for milk-shakes! Put fresh yoghurt and fruit into a blender or food processor with water and sweetening to taste; blend well. Fruits that are particularly nice are bananas and mangoes.

Fresh juices: Freshly prepared fruit or vegetable juice is very nutritious and cleansing. For most fruits and vegetables you will need a proper juicer. However, you can hand squeeze citrus fruit; and white radish/Chinese turnip can be grated and squeezed through muslin. Take once or more during the day.

BEDTIME

If you like, hot milk with ginger, turmeric and ghee (with sugar and cardamom to taste) can be taken at bed-time. This is especially suitable if you have taken a very light evening meal, or are still hungry; eating anything else now will interfere with the quality of your sleep.

REFERENCES

INTRODUCTION

1 Rozenbaum, H, 'European Epidemiology and Society of the menopause', *J Med Assoc Thai*, 81, 1998, Suppl 1: S18.
2 Lazarou, J et al, 'Incidence of adverse drug reactions in hospitalised patients', *Journal of the American Medical Association*, Vol 279, 1998: 1200–5.
3 Classen, D C et al, 'Adverse drug events in hospitalized patients', *Journal of the American Medical Association*, 277 (4) 22/29 Jan 1997: 301–6.
4 Jones, F A, 'New concepts in human nutrition in the twentieth century: The special role of micro-nutrients', *Journal of Nutritional Medicine*, 4, 1994: 99–113.
5 Epstein, S, Chairman of the Cancer Protection Coalition addressing the Neways Convention in Nashville, Tennessee, Jan 1998.
6 Kato, I et al, 'Relationship between westernisation of dietary habits and mortality from breast and ovarian cancer in Japan', *Jpn Journal of Cancer Res*, 78, 1987: 349–57.
7 Newth, K, 'Water Standards Lacking', *Sunday Star Times*, 27 Sept 1998: A 3.

CHAPTER ONE The Mid-life Challenge

1 Sheehy, G, *New Passages*, HarperCollins, 1995: 183–207.
2 Northrup, C, *Women's Bodies, Women's Wisdom*, Bantam, 1995: 435.
3 Beyenne, Y, 'Cultural significance and physical manifestations of menopause, a biocultural analysis', *Cult Med Soc*, 10, 1986: 47–71 cited in Hunter M S, 'Depression and the menopause', *British Medical Journal*, 313, 1996: 1217.
4 Flint, M, 'The menopause: reward or punishment?' *Psychosomatics*, 16, 1975: 161–3 cited in ibid.
5 Tlou, S D, 'The experience of the perimenopause among Botswana women', *University of Illinois at Chicago, Health Sciences Center*, PhD thesis, 1990: 166.
6 Lemke, B, 'Western women and menopause health, quality of life and sexuality', First Asian European Congress on the Menopause, Bangkok, Thailand, Jan 1998.
7 *The Time of our Lives*, A study of mid-life women, 1988, published by Christchurch branch of Society for Research on Women in New Zealand (Inc).

8. Wallace, R K et al, 'The effects of the Transcendental Meditation and TM-Sidhi Program on the aging process', *International Journal of Neuroscience*, 16, 1982: 53–8.
9. Chopra, D, *Ageless Body, Timeless Mind*, Rider, 1993.
10. Gullette, E C D et al, 'Effects of mental stress on myocardial ischemia during daily life', *Journal of the American Medical Association*, 277, 1997: 1521–6.
11. Shinton, R and Sagar, G, 'Lifelong exercise and stroke', *British Medical Journal*, 307, 1993: 231–4.
12. Thune, I et al, 'Physical activity and the risk of breast cancer', *New England Journal of Medicine*, 336, 1997: 1269–75.
13. Wallace, R K et al, ibid.
14. Darrach, B, 'The War on Aging', *Life*, October 1992.
15. Walford, R L, 'The clinical promise of diet restriction', *Geriatrics*, 45 (4) 1990: 81–3, 86–7.

CHAPTER TWO Menopause

1. Pearce, M J and Hawton, K, 'Psychological and sexual aspects of the menopause and HRT', *Baillieres Clin Obstet Gynaecol*, 10 (3) 1996: 385–99.
2. Dennerstein, L, 'Well-being, symptoms and the menopause transition', *Maturitas*, 23 (2) 1996: 147–57.
3. Carranza, L S et al, 'Changes in symptomology, hormones, lipids, and bone density after hysterectomy', *International Journal of Fertility and Women's Medicine*, 42 (1) 1997: 43–7.
4. Matthews, K A, Wing, R R and Kuller, L H, 'Influences of natural menopause on psychological characteristics and symptoms of middle-aged healthy women', *J Consult Clin Psychol*, 58, 1990: 345–63.
5. Avis, N E et al, 'A longitudinal analysis of the association between menopause and depression', *Ann Epidemiol*, 1994: 214–20.
6. Hunter, M S, 'The SE England longitudinal study of the climacteric and postmenopause', *Maturitas*, 14, 1992: 117–26.
7. *The Time of our Lives*, a study of mid-life women, 1988, published by Christchurch Branch of the Society for Research on Women in New Zealand (Inc).
8. Sheehy, G, *New Passages*, Harper Collins, 1995: 183–207.
9. Wolfe, A, 'Menopause: disease or natural changes in life?', First Asian European Congress on the Menopause, Bangkok, Thailand, Jan 1998.
10. Kaufert, 1996, according to Wolfe, A, First Asian European Congress on the Menopause, Bangkok, Thailand, Jan 1998.
11. Win-whe, K, 'Confucian ideology and women's life after menopause', First Asian European Congress on the Menopause, Bangkok, Thailand, Jan 1998.
12. Takumi, Y, 'Oriental medicine in Japan', First Asian European Congress on the Menopause, Bangkok, Thailand, Jan 1998.
13. Hulley, S et al, 'Randomized trial of estrogen plus progestin for secondary prevention of coronary heart disease in postmenopausal women. Heart and Estrogen/progestin Replacement Study (HERS) Research Group', *Journal of the American Medical Association*, 280 (7) 1998: 605–13.
14. Grady, D and Ernster, V 'Hormone replacement therapy and endometrial cancer: Are current regimens safe?', *Journal of National Cancer Inst*, 89 (15) 1997: 1088–9.
15. Grodstein, F, Stampfer, M J and Colditz, G A, 'Postmenopausal hormone therapy and mortality', *New England Journal of Medicine*, 336, 1997: 1769–75.
16. Collaborative Group on Hormonal Factors in Breast Cancer, 'Breast cancer and hormone replacement therapy: Collaborative reanalysis of data from 51 epidemiological studies of 52,705 women with breast cancer and 108,411 women without breast cancer', *Lancet*, 350, 1997: 1047–59.

CHAPTER THREE Ancient Wisdom

1. Lonsdorf, N, *A Woman's Best Medicine*, Tarcher Putnam, 1993: 16.

2 Lumsden, D B et al, 'T'ai chi for osteoarthritis: An introduction for primary care physicians', *Geriatrics*, 53, 1998: 84–8.
3 Uhlmann, R P, 'Tai chi and health', *British Columbia Medical Journal*, 39, 1997: 246–7.
4 Sharma, H M et al, 'Inhibition of human LDL oxidation in vitro by Maharishi Ayur-Veda herbal mixtures', *Pharmacol Biochem Behav*, 43, 1992: 1175–82. See also Sharma, H M, *Freedom From Disease*, Veda Publishing, 1993.
5 Miller, L and Miller, B, *Ayur-Veda and Aromatherapy*, Lotus Press, 1995.

CHAPTER FOUR What Have They Done to our Food?

1 White, A M, 'Pesticides in food: NZ worse than US', *Soil & Health*, February/March 1995: 10–13.
2 Ministry of Health, 1990/91 NZ Total Diet Survey, 1995; Food and Drug Administration, 'Pesticide Program', *Journal of AOAC International*, 76, Sept/Oct 1993.
3 Kong Luen Heong, 'Deadly sprays worse than useless', *New Scientist*, 23 Nov 1996: 7.
4 Colborn, T, Dumanoski, D and Myers, J P, *Our Stolen Future*, Abacus, 1997: 248–9.
5 Jones, F A, 'New concepts in human nutrition in the twentieth century: The special role of micro-nutrients', *Journal of Nutritional Medicine*, 4, 1994: 99–113.
6 Olney, J W et al, 'Increasing brain tumor rates. Is there a link with aspartame?' *Journal of Neuropathy and Experimental Neurology*, 55, 1996: 11.
7 Trichopolous, A M D et al, 'Consumption of olive oil and specific food groups in relation to breast cancer risk in Greece', *Journal of the National Cancer Institute*, 87 (2) 1995: 110–16.
8 Willett, W C et al, 'Intake of trans fatty acids and risk of coronary heart disease among women', *Lancet*, 341, 1993: 581–5.
9 Trichopoulous, A et al, ibid.
10 Wagner, W and Nootbaar, U, 'Prophylactic treatment of migraine with gamma-linolenic and alpha-linolenic acids', *Cephalalgia*, 17 (2) 1997: 127–30; discussion: 102.
11 Horrobin, D F, 'Essential fatty acids in the management of impaired nerve function in diabetes', *Diabetes*, 46, Suppl 2, Sep 1977: S90–3.
12 Zurier, R B et al, 'Gamma-linolenic acid treatment of rheumatoid arthritis. A randomized, placebo-controlled trial', *Arthritis Rheum*, 39 (11) 1996: 1808–17.
13 Jiang, W G et al, 'The effects of n-6 polyunsaturated fatty acids on the expression of nm-23 in human cancer cells', *Br J Cancer*, 77 (5) 1998: 731–8.
14 Kruger, M C and Horrobin, D F, 'Calcium metabolism, osteoporosis and essential fatty acids: A review', *Prog Lipid Res*, 36 (2/3) 1997: 131–151.
15 Cleland, L G and James, M J, 'Rheumatoid arthritis and the balance of dietary n-6 and n-3 essential fatty acids', *British Journal of Rheumatology*, 36, 1997: 513–14 (editorial).
16 Broughton, K et al, 'Reduced asthma symptoms with n-3 fatty acid ingestion are related to 5-series leukotriene production', *American Journal of Clinical Nutrition*, 65, 1997: 1011–17.

CHAPTER FIVE Natural Plant Hormones

1 Murkies, A, 'Phytoestrogens. A clinical review', *J Cli Endocrinol Metab*, 83, 1998: 397–403.
2 Aldercreutz, H, 'Western diet and Western diseases; some hormonal and biochemical mechanisms and associations', *Scand J Clin Lab Invest*, 50 (Suppl 210), 1990: 3–23.
3 Albertazzi, P et al, 'The effect of dietary soy supplementation on hot flushes', *Obstet Gynecol*, 91, 1998: 6–11.
4 Gallagher, J C et al, Creighton University, Omaha, 'The effects of soy isoflavone intake on bone metabolism in post-menopausal women', presented to symposium on the role of soy in preventing and treating chronic disease, Brussels, Belgium, 1996.

5. Ingram, D et al, 'Case-control study of phytoestrogens and breast cancer', *Lancet*, 350, 1997: 990–4.
6. Aldercreutz, H, 'Phytoestrogens: Epidemiology and a possible role in cancer protection', *Environ Health Perspect*, 103 (Suppl 7), 1995: 103–12.
7. Anderson, J W et al, 'Meta-analysis of the effects of soy protein intake on serum lipids', *New England Journal of Medicine*, 333, 1995: 276–82 (a meta-analysis of 38 studies).
8. Stephens, F O, 'Phytoestrogens and prostate cancer: Possible preventive role', *Med J Australia*, 167, 1997: 138–9.
9. Cooper, C, Champion, G and Melton, L J, 'Hip fracture in the elderly: A world wide projection', *Osteoporosis Int*, 2, 1992, 285–9.
10. World Health Organization, 'Assessment of fracture risk and its application to screening for postmenopausal osteoporosis', WHO technical report series No. 843, Geneva, Switzerland, 1994: 11–13.
11. Kato, I, Tominaga, S and Kuroishi, T, 'Relationship between westernisation of dietary habits and mortality from breast and ovarian cancer in Japan', *Jpn J Cancer Res*, 78, 1987: 349–57.
12. Aldercreutz, H et al, 'Urinary excretion of isoflavonoid phytoestrogens and endogenous oestrogens in Japanese or oriental women, and in American and Finnish omnivorous women', referred to in *Lancet*, 338, 1992: 1233.
13. Murkies, Alice, 'Phytoestrogens. A clinical review', *J Cli Endocrinol Metab*, 83, 1998: 397–403.
14. Murkies, A, 'Phytoestrogens — what is the current knowledge?', *Aust Fam Physician*, 27 (Suppl 1), 1998: S47–S51.
15. Murkies, A, ibid.
16. Guy, C, 'From Pink Pills to Phytoestrogens', *Women's Health Watch*, Sept/Oct 1998: 4.
17. Pelton, R, *How to Prevent Breast Cancer*, Fireside Books, 1995: 177.
18. Thompson, L U and Lin, Z, 'Phytic acid and minerals: Effects on early markers of risk for mammary and colon carcinogenisis', *Carcinogenisis*, 12 (11) 1991: 2041–5.
19. New Zealand Charter of Health Practitioners, New Zealand Health Survey, 1997.
20. Liske, E, 'Therapeutic efficacy and safety of *Cimicifuga racemosa*', *Advances in Natural Therapy*, 15 (1) 1998: 45–53.
21. Salzgitter-Schaper & Brummer, 'Remifemin™ — active ingredient: *Cimicifuga* fluid extract: A plant based gynecological agent', scientific brochure, July 1997.
22. Liske, E, ibid.
23. Liske, E, Gerhard, I and Wustenburg, P, 'Menopause: herbal combination product for psychovegetative complaints', *TW Gynäkol*, 10, 1997: 172–5.
24. Grieve, M A, *Modern Herbal*, Jonathan Cape Ltd, UK, 1931.
25. Dittmar, F W et al, 'Premenstrual syndrome (PMS): Treated with a phytopharmaceutical', *TW Gynäkol*, 5 (1), 1992: 60–8.
26. Feldmann, H U et al, 'The treatment of corpus luteum insufficiency and premenstrual syndrome: Experience in a multicenter study under practice conditions', *Hygne*, 11 (12) (1990): 421.
27. Foster, S and Chongxi, Y, *Herbal Emissaries — Bringing Chinese Herbs to the West*, Healing Arts Press, Vermont, 1992.
28. Bone, K, *Clinical Applications of Ayurvedic and Chinese Herbs*, Phytotherapy Press, Warwick, 1995.
29. Weed, Susun, *Menopausal Years. The Wise Woman's Way*, Ash Tree Publishing, 1992.
30. Yhee, Y, Korea, speaking at the First Asian European Conference on the Menopause, Bangkok, Thailand, Jan 1998.
31. Kenton, L, *Passage to Power*, Ebury Press, 1995: 305.
32. Stephens, F O, 'Phytoestrogens and prostate cancer: Possible preventive role', *Med J Australia*, 167, 1997: 138–9.

CHAPTER 6 Natural Hormone Replacement

1. Dalton, K, 'Progesterone suppositories and pessarires in the

treament of migraine', *Headache*, 12 (4) 1973: 151–9.
2. Dalton, K, *Premenstrual Syndrome and Progesterone Therapy*, Heinemann, 1977; *The Premenstrual Syndrome*, Group West, 1985.
3. Lee, J R, *What Your Doctor May Not Tell You About Menopause*, Warner Books, 1996: 124.
4. Archives Journal Club, 'Oestrogen replacement therapy and heart disease', a discussion of the PEPI trial 1995, http://www.ama.assn.org/scipubs/journal/archive/womb/vol-1/no-1/jcr.htm.
5. Cowan, L D et al, 'Breast cancer incidence in women with a history of progesterone deficiency', *American Journal of Epidemiology*, 114, 1981: 209–17.
6. Chang, K J et al, 'Influences of percutaneous administration of estradiol and progesterone on human breast epithelial cell cycle in vivo', *Fertility and Sterility*, 63, 1995: 785–91.
7. Schneider, H P G, 'HRT and gynaecologic malignancy: Breast cancer — European Perspectives', First Asian European Congress on the Menopause, Thailand, Jan 1998.
8. Lee, J, 'Osteoporosis reversal: The role of progesterone', *Clinical Nutrition Review*, 10, 1990: 3.
9. Prior, J C, 'Progesterone as a bone trophic hormone', *Endocrine Reviews*, 11, 1990: 2.
10. Lee, J R, *What Your Doctor May Not Tell You About Menopause*, ibid.
11. Skakkebaek, N and Sharpe, R, 'Are oestrogens involved in falling sperm counts and disorders of the male reproductive tract?', *Lancet*, 341, 1993: 1392–5.
12. Colborn, T et al, *Our Stolen Future*, Abacus, 1997, 66–67.
13. Ilyia, E et al, 'Topical progesterone cream application and overdosing', 4 (1) 1998: 5–6 (letter).
14. Sharma, H, *Freedom from Disease*, Veda Publishing, 1993: 190.
15. Tenover, J S, 'Effects of testosterone supplementation in the aging male', *Journal of Clinical Endocrinological Metabolism*, 75, 1990: 1092–5.
16. Baulieu, E, 'Dehydroepiandrosterone (DHEA): A fountain of youth?' *Journal of Clinical Endocrinology and Metabolism*, 81 (9) 1996: 3147–51.
17. Bates, B, 'Benefit from DHEA not too far fetched', *Family Practice News*, 1 June 1998: 21.
18. Labrie, F et al, 'Effect of 12-month dehydroepiandrosterone replacement therapy on bone, vagina, and endometrium in postmenopausal women', *Journal of Clinical Endocrinology and Metabolism*, 82, 1997: 3498–505.
19. Bates, B, 'Libido decline may signal low testosterone', *Family Practice News*, 15 July 1997: 40.
20. Glaser, J L et al, 'Elevated serum dehydroepiandrosterone sulfate levels in practitioners of the Transcendental (TM) and TM Sidhi programs', *Journal of Behavioural Medicine*, 15 (4), 1992: 327–41.
21. Liebmann, P M et al, 'Melatonin and the immune system', *International Archives of Allergy and Immunology*, 112, 1997: 203–11.
22. Avery, D et al, 'Guidelines for prescribing melatonin', *Annals of Medicine*, 30, 1998: 122–30.
23. Waalen, J, 'Nighttime light studied as possible breast cancer risk', *Journal of the National Cancer Insitute*, 85 (21), 1993: 1712–13.
24. Tan, D et al, 'Melatonin: A potent, endogenous hydroxyl radical scavenger', *Endocrine Journal*, 1, 1993: 57–60.

CHAPTER SEVEN Osteoporosis

1. Spector, T D and Sambrook, P N, 'Steroid osteoporosis', *British Medical Journal*, 307, 1993: 519–20.
2. Buckley, L M et al, 'Calcium and vitamin D-3 supplementation prevents bone loss in spine secondary to low-dose corticosteroids in patients with rheumatoid arthritis', *Annals of Internal Medicine*, 125, 1996: 961–8.
3. Birdsall, T C, 'Prevention of corticosteroid-induced osteoporosis', *Annals of Internal Medicine*, 127, 1997: 90 (letter to the editor).
4. Schneider, D L et al, 'Thyroid hormone use and bone mineral density in elderly women', *Journal of the American Medical Association*, 271 (16) 1994: 1245–9.

5. Hopper, J L and Seeman, E, 'The bone density of female twins discordant for tobacco use', *New England Journal of Medicine*, 330 (6) 1994: 387–92.
6. 'Carbonated beverage and bone fracture in adolescent girls', *American Family Physician*, 50, 1994: 830.
7. *New Zealand Herald*, 5 April 1998, reporting on a study by Reid, I R et al, published in the *Health Research Council Newsletter*, March 1998.
8. Farmer, M E et al, 'Race and sex differences in hip fracture incidence', *American Journal of Public Health*, 74, 1984: 1374–80.
9. Owen, R A et al, 'The national cost of acute care of hip fracture associated with osteoporosis', *Clinical Orthopedics*, 150, 1980: 175.
10. The John R Lee MD (on-line) Medical Letter, October 1998, Website: http://www.johnleemd.com.
11. Sharma, H, *Freedom From Disease*, Veda Publishing, 1993: 93.
12. Abraham, G E, 'The importance of magnesium in the management of primary postmenopausal osteoporosis', *Journal of Nutritional Medicine*, 2, 1991: 165–78.
13. Erdman, J W et al, 'Short term effects of soybean isoflavones on bone in postmenopausal women' (University of Illinois), Second international symposium on the role of soy in preventing and treating disease, Brussels, 1996.
14. Levenson, D I and Bockman, R S, 'A review of calcium preparations' (79 references), *Nutrition Reviews*, 52 (7) 1994: 221–32.
15. Reid, I R et al, 'Effect of calcium supplementation on bone loss in postmenopausal women', *The New England Journal of Medicine*, 328 (7) 1993: 460–4.
16. Heanet, R P, 'Thinking straight about calcium', *The New England Journal of Medicine*, 328 (7) 1993: 503–5.
17. O'Brien, K O, 'Combined calcium and vitamin D supplementation reduces bone loss and fracture incidence in older men and women', *Nutrition Reviews*, 56, May 1998: 148–58.
18. Dreosti, I E, 'Magnesium status and health', *Nutrition Reviews*, 53 (7) 1995: S23–S27.
19. Okano, T, 'Effects of essential trace elements on bone turnover – in relation to osteoporosis', *Nippon Rinsho*, 54 (1) 1996: 148–54.
20. Neilson, F H et al, 'Effect of dietary boron on mineral, estrogen and testosterone metabolism in postmenopausal women', *Federation of Amer Socs for Experimental Biology (FASEB)*, 1, 1987: 394–7.
21. Neer, R M et al, 'Calcitrol or calcium for postmenopausal osteoporosis', *New England Journal of Medicine*, 327 (4) 1992: 357–61, 406–7.
22. Kruger, M C and Horrobin, D, 'Calcium metabolism, osteoporosis and essential fatty acids: A review', *Prog Lipid Res*, 36 (2/3) 1997: 131–51.
23. Michaelsson, K et al, 'Hormone replacement therapy and the risk of hip fracture: population based cars-controlled study', *British Medical Journal*, 316, 1998: 1858–63.
24. Khaw, K, 'Hormone replacement therapy again', *British Medical Journal*, 316, 1998: 1842–4.
25. Lee, J R, 'Osteoporosis reversal: the role of progesterone', *International Clinical Nutrition Review*, 10 (3) 1990: 384–91.
26. Prior, J C, 'Progesterone as a bone-trophic hormone', *Endocrine Reviews*, 11 (2) 1990: 386–90.
27. Lee, J R, 'Osteoporosis reversal with transdermal progesterone' (letter), *Lancet*, 336, 1990: 1327.
28. Labrie, F et al, 'Effect of 12-month dehydroepiandrosterone replacement therapy on bone, vagina, and endometrium in postmenopausal women', *Journal of Clinical Endocrinology and Metabolism*, 82, 1997: 3498–505.

CHAPTER EIGHT Breast Cancer

1. Colditz, G A et al, 'Family history, age, and risk of breast cancer', *Journal of the American Medical Association*, 270 (3) 1993: 338–43.
2. Ibid.
3. Ibid.

4 Ibid.
5 Malone, K E et al, 'Family history and survival of young women with invasive breast carcinoma', *Cancer*, 78 (7) 1996: 1417–25.
6 MacMahon, B et al, 'Age at First Birth and Breast Cancer Risk', World Health Organisation Bulletin 43, 1970: 209–21.
7 Malins, D C et al, 'Progression of human breast cancers to the metastatic state is linked to hydroxyl radical-induced DNA damage', Proceedings of the National Academy of Sciences USA, 93 (6) 1996: 2557–63.
8 Wolk, A et al, 'A prospective study of association of monounsaturated fat and other types of fat with risk of breast cancer', *Archives of Internal Medicine*, 158, 1998: 41–5.
9 Smith, W S A et al (Department of Nutrition, Harvard School of Public Health, Boston, Mass), 'Alcohol and breast cancer in women: A pooled analysis of cohort studies', *Journal of the American Medical Association*, 279 (7) 1998: 535–40.
10 Plu Bureau, G et al, 'Oral contraception and the risk of breast cancer', *Contracept Fertil Sex*, 25 (4) 1997: 301–5.
11 Collaborative Group on Hormonal Factors in Breast Cancer, 'Breast cancer and hormone replacement therapy: Collaborative reanalysis of data from 51 epidemiological studies of 52,705 women with breast cancer and 108,411 women without breast cancer', *Lancet*, 350, 1997: 1047–59.
12 Collaborative Group on Hormonal Factors in Breast Cancer, ibid, discussed by Charlotte Paul in *Women's Health Update*, Jan 1998.
13 Wartenburg, D and Stapleton, C, 'Risk of Breast Cancer is also increased among retired U.S. female airline cabin attendants' (letter), *British Medical Journal*, 316, 1998: 1902.
14 Bennicke, K et al, 'Cigarette smoking and breast cancer', *British Medical Journal*, 310, 1995: 1431–3.
15 Glasziou, P P et al, 'Mammogaphic screening trials for women aged under 50', *The Medical Journal of Australia*, 162, 1995: 625–9.
16 Wright, C and Mueller, C, 'Screening and mammography and public health policy: The need for perspective', *Lancet*, 346, 1995: 29–32.
17 Porfiri, L M et al, 'A mammographic evaluation of the morphostructural variations of the breast during hormone-replacement therapy in the postmenopause', *Radiol Med (Torino)*, 95 (6) 1998: 573–6.
18 Elmore, J G et al, 'Ten-year risk of false positive screening mammograms and clinical breast exams', *New England Journal of Medicine*, 338, 1998: 1089–96.
19 Cuzick, J et al, 'Electropotential measurements as a new diagnostic modality for breast cancer', *Lancet*, 352, 1998: 359–63.
20 Randal, J, 'Heat-seeking pads may help to find early breast cancers', *Journal of the National Cancer Institute*, 89, 1 October 1997: 1402–4.
21 Ingram, D et al, 'Case-control study of phyto-oestrogens and breast cancer', *Lancet*, 350, 1997: 990–4.
22 Messina, M et al, 'Phyto-oestrogens and breast cancer', *Lancet*, 350, 1997: 971–2.
23 Imai, K et al, 'Cancer-preventive effects of drinking green tea among a Japanese population', *Preventive Medicine*, 26, November/December 1997: 769–75.
24 Wolk, A et al, ibid.
25 Trichopolous, A M D et al, 'Consumption of olive oil and specific food groups in relation to breast cancer risk in Greece', *Journal of the National Cancer Institute*, 87 (2) 1995: 110–16.
26 Bougnoux, P et al, 'Alpha linolenic acid content of adipose breast tissue: A host determinant of the risk of early metastasis in breast cancer', *British Journal of Cancer*, 70 (2) 1994: 330–4.
27 Jain, M et al, 'Premorbid diet and the prognosis of women with breast cancer', *Journal of the National Cancer Institute*, 86 (18) 1994: 1390–7.
28 Sharma, H M et al, 'Inhibition of human LDL oxidation in vitro by Moharishi Ayur-Veda herbal mixtures', *Pharmacol Biochem Behav*, 43, 1992: 1175–82. Refer D R Hari Sharma's book *Freedom From Disease*, Veda Publishing, 1993.

29. Turley, J M et al, 'Vitamin E succinate induces Fas-mediated apopyosis in estrogen receptor-negative human breast cancer cells', *Cancer Research*, 57, 1997: 881–90.
30. Willett, W C, 'Micronutrients and cancer risk', *American Journal of Clinical Nutrition*, 59 (Suppl), May 1994: 1162S–65S.
31. Larsen, H R, 'Coenzyme Q10: The wonder nutrient', *Int Journ Alt and Comp Medicine*, 16 (2) 1998: 11–12.
32. Clark, L C et al, 'Effects of selenium supplementation for cancer prevention in patients with carcinoma of the skin', *Journal of the American Medical Association*, 276 (24) 1996: 1957–63.
33. Colditz, G A, 'Selenium and cancer prevention — promising results indicate further trials required', *Journal of the American Medical Association*, 276 (24) 1996: 1984–5 (editorial).
34. 'Auckland top of list in toxic air' by Philip English, *New Zealand Herald*, 1 October 1998: A7.
35. Hunter, D J et al, 'Plasma organochlorine levels and the risk of breast cancer', *New England Journal of Medicine*, 337, 1997: 1253–8.
36. Manz, A et al, 'Cancer mortality among workers in a chemical plant contaminated with dioxin', *Lancet*, 338, 1991: 959–64.
37. Westin, J B and Richter, E, 'The Israeli breast cancer anomaly', *Annals of the New York Academy of Sciences*, 609, 1990: 269–79.
38. Epstein, S and Steinman, D, *The Breast Cancer Prevention Program*, Macmillan Publishing, Indianapolis, 1998.
39. Lemus-Wilson, A et al, 'Melatonin blocks the stimulatory effects of prolactin on human breast cancer cell growth in culture', *British Journal of Cancer*, 72 (6) 1995: 1435–40.
40. Stevens, R G and Davis, S, 'The melatonin hypothesis: Electric power and breast cancer', *Environ Health Perspect*, 104 (Suppl 1) 1996: 135–40.
41. Murch, S J et al, 'Melatonin in feverfew and other medicinal plants', *Lancet*, 350 (9091) 1997: 1598–9.
42. Blask, D E et al, 'Physiological melatonin inhibition of human breast cancer cell growth in vitro: Evidence for a glutathione mediated pathway', *Cancer Research*, 57, 1997: 1909–14.
43. Cowan, L D et al, 'Breast cancer incidence in women with a history of progesterone deficiency', *American Journal of Epidemiology*, 114, 1981: 209–17.
44. Schneider, H P G, 'HRT and gynaecologic malignancy: Breast cancer — European perspectives', First Asian European Congress on the Menopause, Thailand, Jan 1998.
45. Chang, K J et al, 'Influences of percutaneous administration of estradiol and progesterone on human breast epithelial cell cycle in vivo', *Fertility and Sterility*, 63, 1995: 785–91.
46. Mohr, P E et al, 'Serum progesterone and prognosis in operable breast cancer', *British Journal of Cancer*, 73 (12) 1996: 1552–5.
47. Thune, I et al, 'Physical activity and the risk of breast cancer', *New England Journal of Medicine*, 336, 1997: 1269–75.
48. Flach, J and Seachrist, L, 'Mind-body meld may boost immunity', *Journal of the National Cancer Institute*, 86 (4) 1994: 256–8.
49. Levy, S et al, 'Survival hazards analysis in first recurrence breast cancer patients; seven-year follow-up', *Psychosomatic Med*, 50, 1988: 520–8.
50. Eppley, K et al, 'Differential effects of relaxation techniques on trait anxiety; a meta-analysis', *Journal of Clinical Psychology*, 45, 1989: 957–74.
51. Orme-Johnson, D W, 'Medical care and the transcendental meditation program', *Psychosomatic Medicine*, 49, 1987: 493–507.
52. Chang, S, Chang, R and Harvey, A, 'Perineal talc exposure and risk of ovarian carcinoma', *Cancer*, 79, 1997: 2396–401.

CHAPTER NINE Women and Heart Disease

1. Nyyssonen, K et al, 'Vitamin C

deficiency and risk of myocardial infarction: Prospective population study of men from eastern Finland', *British Medical Journal*, 314, 1997: 634–8.
2 Enstrom, J E, 'Vitamin C intake and mortality among a sample of the United States population', *Epidemiology*, 3, 1992: 194–202.
3 Bendich, A et al, 'Potential health economic benefits of vitamin supplementation', *Western Journal of Medicine*, 166, 1997: 306–12.
4 Stampfer, M J et al, 'Vitamin E consumption and the risk of coronary disease in women and men', *New England Journal of Medicine*, 328 (20) 1993: 1444–56.
5 Sharma, H, *Freedom from Disease*, Veda Publishing, Toronto: 126.
6 Larsen, H R, 'Coenzyme Q10: The wonder nutrient', *Int Journ Alt and Comp Medicine*, 16 (2) 1998: 11–12.
7 Rimm, E B et al, 'Folate and vitamin B-6 from diet and supplements in relation to risk of coronary heart disease among women', *Journal of the American Medical Association*, 279, 1998: 359–64.
8 McCully, K S, 'Homocysteine, folate, vitamin B-6, and cardiovascular disease', *Journal of the American Medical Association*, 279, 1998: 392–3 (editorial).
9 Philip, C S, 'Effect of niacin supplementation on fibrinogen levels in patients with peripheral vascular disease', *American Journal of Cardiology*, 82, 1998: 697–9.
10 Niwa, J, 'Effect of Maharishi-4 and Maharishi-5 on inflammatory mediators — with special reference to their free radical scavenging effect', *Indian Journal of Clinical Practice*, 1, 1991: 23–7.
11 Tomlinson, P F Jr and Wallace, R K, *Journal Fed Am Soc Exper Biol*, 5, 1991: A1284 (Abstract); refer Sharma's book (below).
12 Sharma, H M et al, *Pharmacol Biochem Behav*, 43, 1992: 1175–82; refer Sharma's book *Freedom From Disease*, Veda Publishing, 1993.
13 Reusser, M E and McCarron, D A, 'Micronutrient effects on blood pressure regulation', *Nutrition Reviews*, 52 (11) 1994: 367–75.
14 Reusser, M E and McCarron, D A, ibid.
15 Trichopolous, A M D et al, 'Consumption of olive oil and specific food groups in relation to breast cancer risk in Greece', *Journal of the National Cancer Institute*, 87 (2) 1995: 110–16.
16 Hulley, S et al, Heart and Estrogen/Progestin Replacement Study (HERS) Research Group, 'Randomized trial of estrogen plus progestin for secondary prevention of coronary heart disease in postmenopausal women', *Journal of the American Medical Association*, 280 (7) 1998: 605–13.
17 Gullette, E C D et al, 'Effects of mental stress on myocardial ischemia during daily life', *Journal of the American Medical Association*, 277, (20) 1997: 1521–6.
18 Kubzansky, L D et al, 'Is worrying bad for your heart? A prospective study of worry and coronary heart disease in the Normative Aging Study', *Circulation*, 95 (4) 1997: 818–24.
19 Orme-Johnson, D W, 'Medical care utilisation and the transcendental meditation program', *Psychosomatic Medicine*, 49, 1987: 493–507.
20 Hakim, A A et al, 'Effects of walking on mortality among nonsmoking retired men', *New England Journal of Medicine*, 338, 1998: 94–9.
21 Stefanick, M L et al, 'Effects of diet and exercise in men and post-menopausal women with low levels of HDL cholesterol and high levels of LDL cholesterol', *New England Journal of Medicine*, 399 (1) 1998: 12–20

CHAPTER TEN Depression

1 Matthews, K A, Wing, R R and Kuller, L H, 'Influences of natural menopause on psychological characteristics and symptoms of middle-aged healthy women', *J Consult Clin Psychol*, 58, 1990: 345–63.
2 Avis, N E, Brambilla, D, McKinlay, S M and Vass, K, 'A longitudinal analysis of the association between menopause and depression', *Ann Epidemiol*, 4, 1994: 214–20.

3. Hunter, M S, 'The SE England longitudinal study of the climacteric and postmenopause', *Maturitas*, 14, 1992: 117–26.
4. Nicol-Smith, L, 'Causality, menopause, and depression: A critical review of the literature', *British Medical Journal*, 313, 1996: 1229–32.
5. Northrup, C, *Women's Bodies, Women's Wisdom*, Bantam, 1995: 460.
6. Carranza, L S et al, 'Changes in symptomology, hormones, lipids, and bone density after hysterectomy', *International Journal of Fertility and Women's Medicine*, 42 (1) 1997: 43–7.
7. Woeber, K A, 'Subclinical thyroid dysfunction', *Archives of Internal Medicine*, 157, 1997: 1065–8.
8. Siblerud, R L et al, 'Psychometric evidence that dental amalgam mercury may be an etiological factor in manic depression', *Journal of Orthomolecular Medicine*, 13 (1) 1998: 31–40.
9. Siblerud, R L and Kienholz, E, 'Evidence that mercury from dental amalgam may cause hearing loss in multiple sclerosis patients', *Journal of Orthomolecular Medicine*, 12 (4) 1997: 240–4.
10. Bloomfield, H et al, *Hypericum (St John's wort) and Depression*, Prelude Press, 1997.
11. Upton, R et al, 'St John's wort *Hypericum perforatum*: Quality control, analytical and therapeutic monograph', *American Herbal Pharmacopoeia and Therapeutic Compendium*, July 1997: 1–32 and references therein.
12. De Smet, P A and Nolen, W A, 'St John's wort as an antidepressant', *British Medical Journal*, 313 (7052) 1996: 241–7.
13. Linde, K et al, 'St John's wort for depression — an overview and meta-analysis of randomised clinical trials', *British Medical Journal*, 313 (7052) 1996: 253–8.
14. Anon, 'Herbal treatment for depression: launch of St John's wort study', *The Herbal Doctor* (the official newsletter of the Australian College of Herbal Medicine), 1 (1) 1997: 2.
15. Volz, H P, 'Long-term kava therapy for anxiety', Sixth Phytotherapy Conference, Berlin, 1995.
16. Eppley, K et al, 'Differential effects of relaxation techniques on trait anxiety; a meta-analysis', *Journal Clin Psychol*, 45, 1989: 957–74.
17. Liske, E, Gerhard, I and Wustenburg, P, 'Menopause: herbal combination product for psychovegetative complaints', *TW Gynäkol*, 10, 1997: 172–5.

CHAPTER ELEVEN Minerals

1. Cited in: Sharma H, *Freedom from Disease*, Veda Publishing, 1993: 117.
2. Clark, L C et al, 'Effects of selenium supplementation for cancer prevention in patients with carcinoma of the skin', *Journal of the American Medical Association*, 276 (24) 1996: 1957–63.
3. Colditz, G A, 'Selenium and cancer prevention — promising results indicate further trials required', *Journal of the American Medical Association*, 276 (24), 1996: 1984–5 (editorial).
4. Singh, R B et al, 'Magnesium status and risk of coronary artery disease in rural and urban populations with variable magnesium consumption', *Magnes Res*, 10 (3) 1997: 205–13.
5. *American Heart Journal*, October 1992: 1113–18.
6. Yusuf, S et al, 'Intravenous magnesium in acute myocardial infarction', *Circulation*, 87, 1993: 2043–6.
7. Woods, K L and Fletcher, S, 'Long-term outcome after intravenous magnesium sulphate in suspected acute myocardial infarction: the second Leicester Intravenous Magnesium Intervention Trial' (LIMIT-2), *Lancet*, 343, 1994: 816–19.
8. Dreosti, I E, 'Magnesium status and health', *Nutrition Reviews*, 53 (9) 1995: S23–7.
9. Keenan, J M and Morris, D H, 'How to make sure your older patients are getting enough zinc', *Geriatrics*, 48 (10) 1993: 57–65.

REFERENCES

10 Boukaiba, N, 'A physiological amount of zinc supplementation: Effects on nutritional. lipid, and thymic status in an elderly population', *American Journal of Clinical Nutrition*, 57, 1993: 566–72.
11 Mossad, S B et al, 'Zinc gluconate lozenges for treating the common cold', *Annals of Internal Medicine*, 125 (2) 1996: 81–8.
12 Sandstead, H H, 'Requirements and toxicity of essential trace elements, illustrated by zinc and copper', *American Journal of Clinical Nutrition*, 61 (3) 1995: 621S–624S.
13 Wood, R J and Zheng, J J, 'High dietary calcium intakes reduce zinc absorption and balance in humans', *American Journal of Nutrition*, 65, 1997: 1803–9.
14 Abraham, A S, 'The effects of chromium supplementation on serum glucose and lipids in patients with and without non-insulin dependent diabetes', *Metabolism*, 41 (7) 1992: 768–71 (as cited in Carper, J, *Stop Ageing Now!*, Thorsons, 1997).
15 Mertz, W, 'Chromium in human nutrition: A review', *Journal of Nutrition*, 123, April 1993: 626–33.
16 Abraham, A S, ibid.
17 Evans, G W, 'Chromium picolinate increases longevity', *Age*, 15, 1992: 134 (abstract).
18 Thomson, C D and Robinson, M F, 'The changing selenium status of New Zealand residents', *Eur J Clin Nutr*, 50 (2) 1996: 107–14.
19 Clark, L C et al, ibid.
20 Colditz, G A, ibid.
21 Giovannucci, E, 'Selenium and risk of prostate cancer', *Lancet*, 352 (9130) 1998: 755–6.
22 Han, Jui, 'Highlights of the cancer chemoprevention studies in China', *Preventive Medicine*, 22, 1993: 712–22.
23 Delmas-Beauvieux, M et al, 'The enzymatic antioxidant system in blood and glutathione status in human immunodeficiency virus (HIV)-infected patients: Effects of supplementation with selenium or beta-carotene', *American Journal of Clinical Nutrition*, 64, 1996: 101–7.
24 *American Journal of Clinical Nutrition*, April 1992: 885–90.
25 Goyer, R A, 'Nutrition and metal toxicity', *American Journal of Clinical Nutrition*, 61 (3) 1995: 646S–650S.

CHAPTER TWELVE Secrets of a Long and Healthy Life

1 Frentzel-Beyme, R and Chang-Claude, J, 'Vegetarian diets and colon cancer: The German experience', *American Journal of Clinical Nutrition*, 59, May 1994: 1143S–52S (suppl).
2 Epstein, S, Chairman of the Cancer Prevention Coalition, addressing the Neways Convention, Nashville in Tennessee, Jan 1998.
3 English, P, 'Auckland top of list in toxic air', *New Zealand Herald*, 1 October 1998: A7.
4 Cousins, N, *Anatomy of an Illness*, Bantam, 1991.
5 Greer, S, 'Psychological response to cancer and survival', *Psychological Medicine*, 21, 1991: 43–9. Cited in Pecton, R et al, *How to Prevent Breast Cancer*, Simon & Schuster, 1995: 284.
6 Willich, S N et al, 'Weekly variation of acute myocardial infarction', *Circulation*, 90 (1) 1994: 87–93.
7 Kubzansky, L D et al, 'Is worrying bad for your heart? A prospective study of worry and coronary heart disease in the Normative Aging Study', *Circulation*, 95 (4) 1997: 818–24.
8 Felitti, V J et al, 'Relationship of childhood abuse and household dysfunction to many of the leading causes of death in adults', *American Journal of Preventive Medicine*, 14, May 1998: 245–58.
9 Weiss, M J S and Wagner, S H, 'What explains the negative consequences of adverse childhood experiences on adult health?', *American Journal of Preventive Medicine*, 14, May 1998: 356–60 (commentary).
10 Shinton, R and Sagar, G, 'Lifelong exercise and stroke', *British Medical Journal*, 307, 1993: 231–4.
11 Thune, I et al, 'Physical activity and the risk of breast cancer', *New England Journal of Medicine*, 336, 1997: 1269–75.

12 Chopra, D, *Ageless Body, Timeless Mind*, Rider, 1993: 86.
13 Fiatarone, M A, 'Exercise training and nutritional supplementation for physical frailty in very elderly people', *The New England Journal of Medicine*, 330 (25) 1994: 1769–75.
14 CNN, *Science Daily*, reported in *Partners*, the AIM news magazine, 6 (7) 1998 (AIM is an International multi-level marketing co).
15 Coney, S, *Feeling Fabulous at 40, 50 and Beyond*, Tandem, 1996: 122.
16 Hakim, A A et al, 'Effects of walking on mortality among nonsmoking retired men', *New England Journal of Medicine*, 338, 1998: 94–9.
17 Sharma, H, *Freedom from Disease*, Veda Publishing, 1993: 173.
18 Eppley, K et al, 'Differential effects of relaxation techniques on trait anxiety: a meta-analysis', *Journal Clin Psych*, 45, 1989: 957–74.
19 Orme-Johnson, D W, 'Medical care utilisation and the transcendental meditation program', *Psychosomatic Medicine*, 49, 1987: 493–507.

CHAPTER 13 Natural Solutions

1 Liske, E, Gerhard, I and Wustenburg, P, 'Menopause: Herbal combination product for psychovegetative complaints', *TW Gynäkol*, 10, 1997: 172–5.
2 Eppely, K et al, 'Differential effects of relaxation techniques on trait anxiety: a meta-analysis', *Journal Clin Psychol*, 45, 1989: 957–74.
3 Magee, E, *Eat Well for a Healthy Menopause*, Wiley, 1996: 32.
4 Perrig, W J et al, 'The relation between antioxidants and memory performance in the old and very old', *Journal of the American Geriatrics Society*, 45, 1997: 718–24.
5 Le Bars, P L et al, 'A placebo-controlled, double-blind, randomized trial of an extract of ginkgo biloba for dementia', *Journal of the American Medical Association*, 278, 1997: 1327–32.
6 Sano, M et al, 'A controlled trial of selegiline, alpha-tocopherol, or both as treatment for Alzheimer's disease', *New England Journal of Medicine*, 336, 1997: 1216–22.
7 CNN, *Science Daily*, reported in *Partners*, 6 (7) 1998.
8 Wagner, W Nootbaar and Wagner, U, 'Prophylactic treatment of migraine with gamma-linolenic and alpha-linolenic acids', *Cephalalgia*, 17 (2) 1997: 127–30; discussion 102.
9 Lee, J, *What Your Doctor May Not Tell You About Menopause*, Warner books, 1996: 98.
10 Cabot, S, *The Liver Cleansing Diet*, WHAS, 1996.

SUGGESTED READING

Bloomfield, Harold H; McWilliams, Peter, *Hypericum and Depression*, Prelude Press, 1997.

Colborn, Theo; Dumanoski, Dianne; Peterson Myers, John, *Our Stolen Future*, Abacus, 1997.

Coney, Sandra, *Feeling Fabulous at 40, 50 and Beyond*, Tandem, 1996.

Coney, Sandra, *The Menopause Industry*, Penguin, 1992.

Epstein, Samuel, MD, Steinman, David, *The Breast Cancer Prevention Program*, Macmillan, 1998.

Kedgely, Sue, *Eating Safely in a Toxic World*, Penguin, 1998.

Kenton, Leslie, *Passage to Power*, Ebury Press, 1995.

Lee, John, *What Your Doctor May Not Tell You About Menopause*, Warner Books, 1996.

Lonsdorf, Nancy, MD; Butler, Veronica, MD; Brown, Melanie, PhD, *A Woman's Best Medicine: Health, Happiness and Long Life through Maharishi Ayur-Veda*, Tarcher Putnam, 1995.

Northrup, Christiane, MD, *Women's Bodies, Women's Wisdom*, Bantam, 1995.

Pelton, Ross; Clarke Pelton, Taffy; Vint, Vinton, *How to Prevent Breast Cancer*, Fireside, 1995.

Sharma, Hari, MD, *Freedom From Disease*, Veda Publishing, 1993.

Steinman, David; Epstein, Samuel, MD, *The Safe Shopper's Bible, A Consumer's Guide to Non-Toxic Household Products, Cosmetics and Food*, Macmillan, 1995.

Weed, Susun, *Menopausal Years. The Wise Woman's Way*, Ash Tree Publishing, 1992.

SALUTE TO THE SUN (SURYANAMASKAR)

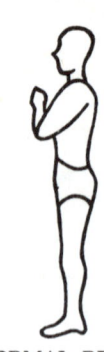

NORMAL, RESTFUL BREATHING
1. Salutation Position

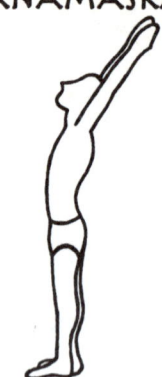

INHALE
2. Raised Arms Position

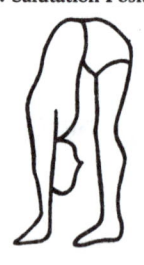

EXHALE
3. Hand to Foot Position

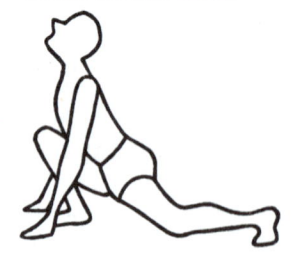

INHALE
4. Equestrian Position

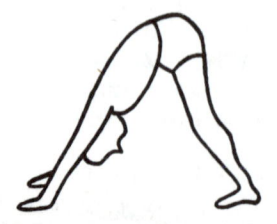

EXHALE
5. Mountain Position

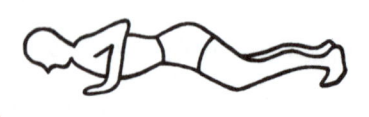

NO BREATHING THEN...
(Number 7)
6. Eight Limbs Position

SALUTE TO THE SUN 223

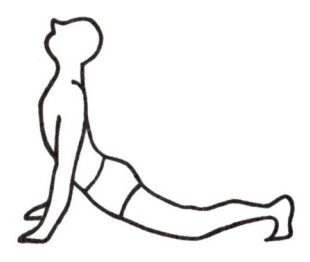

INHALE
7. Cobra Position

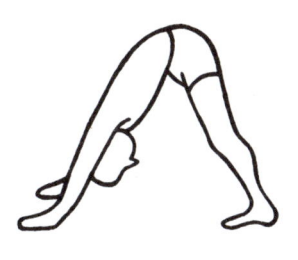

EXHALE
8. Mountain Position

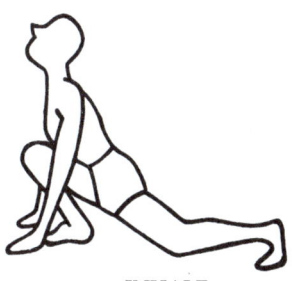

INHALE
9. Equestrian Position

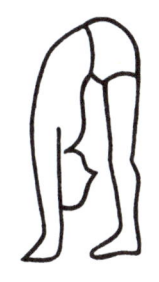

EXHALE
10. Hand to Foot Position

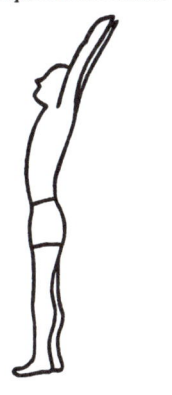

INHALE
11. Raised Arms Position

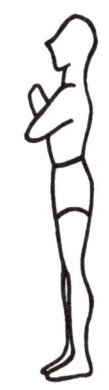

NORMAL, RESTFUL BREATHING
12. Salutation Position

INDEX

ageing 24–8, 172
alcohol 109, 123, 170
Alzheimer's disease 188–9
amalgam 146
antioxidants (*see* vitamins *and* minerals) 29, 77, 128–9, 140, 142
anxiety 156–157, 184
Aspartame (Nutrasweet) 66–7
atherosclerosis 137, 139, 140
Ayur-Veda 44–57, 128, 130, 136–7, 177
  Amrit Kalash 45, 128, 140, 170
  and diet 52–4
  and menopause symptoms 51–2
  body types 47–56
    Kapha 47–56
    Pitta 47–56
    Vata 47–56
  essential oils 55–7
  Maharishi Mahesh Yogi 45
  menopause strategies 51–2
  menopause symptoms 50–1
  treatments 46–7, 54–7

beta-carotene 139
biological age 28
black cohosh 82–3, 158
blood clots 39
breast cancer 39–40, 63, 77–8, 82, 91, 96, 106, 121–134, 173
  alcohol 123
  coenzyme Q10 129, 139
  detection and treatment 124–7
  HRT 124
  polyunsaturated fats 123
  mammography 126
  natural progesterone 132
  oral contraceptives 123
  smoking 124
  sunlight 132
  timing surgery 132

calcium 108–115, 117, 118, 141, 159, 160, 168, 170
cancer
  brain 66
  breast 39–40, 63, 77–8, 82, 91, 96, 106, 121–134, 173
  cervical 106
  colon 77, 168
  endometrial 39
  ovarian 134
  prostate 63, 77, 96
  rectal 168
canola 64, 71
chaste tree 83–8
chemicals 60–1, 62–3, 171–2
  pesticides and herbicides in New Zealand 59–61
  DDT 60, 63, 95–6, 124, 129–31
  PCBs 63, 95–6, 129–31
  thalidomide 60–1
  tryptophan 60–1
cholesterol 68–9, 90, 163, 165, 168
Christiane Northrup, *Women's Bodies, Women's Wisdom* 25, 145
Coca Cola 61
coenzyme Q10 139
Colburn T., Dunanoski D., and Myers J. P., *Our Stolen Future* 60
Coney, Sandra, *Feeling Fabulous at 40, 50 and Beyond* 175–6
Cousins, Norman, *Anatomy of an Illness* 173

DDT (*see* chemicals)
depression (at menopause) 144–57
  and thyroid 146
  physical causes 145–6
  St Johns wort 147–55
  symptoms of 146–7
  treatments for anxiety 156–7
    kava kava 156–7

225

DHEA 103–4, 119, 166
diabetes 61, 160, 163, 166, 174
DNA 13, 63–64, 95–96, 128
dong quai/tang kuei 84–5

endometrial cancer 39
Epstein, Samuel and Steinman, David, *The Breast Cancer Prevention Programme* 131
evening primrose oil (GLA) 72–3, 117
exercise 27, 36, 107, 111, 142, 174–7, 183
  excessive 109–110
fats 68–74
  canola 71
  essential fatty acids 72–7
    alpha-linolenic acid (n-3) 73–4, 127
    linoleic acid (n-6) 72–4
    gamma-linolenic acid (GLA) 72–3
    evening primrose oil 72–3, 117
  margarine 70–1
    'trans' fatty acids 70
  saturated 68–9
    cholesterol 68–9, 90, 163, 165, 168
    high density lipids (HDL) 69, 90, 136
    low density lipids (LDL) 69, 136, 165
  oils 71–2
  olive oil 72, 127
  unsaturated 69–70
    monounsaturates 69–70, 127
    polyunsaturates 69–70, 123, 127
folic acid 139–140
food and diet (*see* nutrition)
free radicals 77, 104, 166, 170–1,
fertility 60, 96–7
free radicals 29, 122–3, 133

gall bladder disease 39, 61

genetic engineering 63–66, 80–1, 131, 170
  canola 64
  DNA 63–4
  gene-altered food labelling 65
  soy 64, 66
ginseng 29, 85

hair mineral analysis 120, 162, 224
headaches 92, 189
heart disease 61, 77, 90–1, 135–43, 171, 173
  and diet 141
  and exercise 142
  and HRT 142
  and stress 142
  atherosclerosis 136, 138, 139
  cholesterol 68–9, 90,163, 168
  high blood pressure 141–2, 163, 168, 173–4
  hypertension 142, 163
herbal medicines 39
hormone replacement therapy (HRT) 35, 39–41, 82, 84, 88, 89, 105, 109, 118, 124, 125, 142
hormones 76–9
  and osteoporosis 117
  DHEA 102–3, 117, 119, 166
  follicle-stimulating hormone (FSH) 93
  HRT 35, 39–41, 82, 84, 88, 89, 105, 109, 118, 124, 125, 142
  human growth hormone 117
  melatonin 102–3, 104
  natural 88–105
  oestrogen 76, 102, 104, 108, 117, 130
  progesterone 38, 88–93, 94, 97–98, 108, 117, 118, 132
  testosterone 102–3
  the role of 131–2
hot flushes 32, 36, 77–8, 82, 83, 86, 182–3
high blood pressure 141–2, 163, 168, 173–4

hypothalamus 38, 93, 94
hysterectomy 36, 145

infertility 63, 96–7
   diethylstilbestrol (DES) 96

Jones, Sir Francis Avery, *Journal of Nutritional Medicine* 61–2

kava kava 156–7
Kedgley, Sue, *Eating Safely in a Toxic World* 65
Kenton, Leslie, *Passage to Power* 87

Lee, Dr John, *What Your Doctor May Not Tell You About Menopause* 90, 100
libido 186
low self-esteem 36

magnesium 108, 112–3, 118, 141, 160, 170
meditation 27, 51, 103–4, 133, 178–9
   Transcendental Meditation 28, 51, 103–4, 133–4, 157, 178–9
menopause 22, 24, 31–41, 77, 89, 122
   approaches to 94
   attitudes to 24–6
   herbs for 82–8
   natural solutions for 181–91
   symptoms of (physical) 32–3
      aching joints 187
      breast tenderness 191
      creepy skin 33–4
      dizziness 83
      dry vagina 83, 185–6
      fatigue 32–3, 190
      fluid retention 191
      headaches 189
      hot flushes 32, 36, 77–8, 82, 83, 86, 182–3
      incontinence/urinary problems 186–7
      menstrual flooding 190
      night sweats 32–3, 86, 182–3
      skin problems 190
      weight gain 190–1
   symptoms of (psychological) 33, 36
      depression 35–6, 83, 86, 144–57, 184–5
      insomnia 184
      loss of libido 33, 186
      memory loss 33–4, 187–8
menstrual cycle 92–4, 122
   corpus luteum 94
   heavy menstrual bleeding 87
   luteinising hormone (LH) 93, 94
   ovulation 93
   premenstrual syndrome (PMS) 84, 89, 92, 96, 163
migraine 90, 163
minerals 107–8, 112–8, 129, 141, 158–68, 170
   calcium 108–115, 117, 118, 141, 159–60, 164, 168, 170
   chromium 160, 165–6
   magnesium 108, 112–3, 118, 141, 160, 162–4, 170
   selenium 129, 159, 166–7, 170
   zinc 115, 160, 164–5
   testing for (hair analysis) 120, 162, 224

night sweats 32–3, 86, 182–3
nutrition 29, 52–3, 58–74, 141, 170–1
   Asian women 39
   history of 61–2
   Japanese women 29

obesity 61
oestrogen 38, 76, 78, 90, 95–97, 108
   dominance of 95, 99
   environmental 95–6
   natural 104–4
oils (*see* fats)
oral contraceptives 123

osteoporosis 77–8, 106–120, 163
  and hormones 117
  causes of 108–11
  drugs 119
  risk factors 108
  testing for 119–20
    Dual Energy X-ray Absorptiometry (DEXA scan) 91, 111, 120
ovulation 93

phytoestrogens (natural plant hormones) 87, 113–4, 126–7
  coumestans 78–9
  foods rich in 81
  isoflavones 78–9
  linseed 76
  lignans 78–9
  saponins 78–9
  supplements 81–2
  vitex agnus castus 76
premenstrual syndrome (PMS) 84, 89, 92, 96, 163
progesterone 38, 89–93, 94, 97–8
  and menopause 91–2
  and osteoporosis 91–2
  and PMS 92
  natural 88–92, 98–9, 118–9, 132
    cream 88–92, 99–100, 118–9
    side-effects 99
  properties of 97–8

red clover 81, 85–6
rheumatoid arthritis 73–4

sage 84–5, 86
salute to the sun (suryanamaskar) 177, 222–3
seaweeds, sea vegetables 112, 163, 168, 170, 196–9
Sharma, Dr Hari, *Freedom from Disease* 177–8

Sheehy, Gail, *New Passages* 22
smoking 109, 124, 135
soy and soy products 64, 77, 79–81, 127
  and infants 79
  genetic engineering of 80
  phytates 80
  protease inhibitors 80
St Johns wort (*hypericum*) 83, 86, 147–55, 157
stress 133–4, 135, 142

T'ai chi 44
thyroid 146
Transcendental Meditation 28, 51, 103–4, 133–4, 157, 178–9
tumours 167

vaginal dryness 32, 39, 185
vegetarians 167, 170–1
vitamins 114–6, 118, 128–9, 137–40, 158, 170, 173
  A 115, 129, 139, 159
  B 139–40
  B_6 116, 139
  C 115, 118, 128, 137, 159, 170, 173
  D 114, 118, 128, 159
  E 128, 138–40, 170
  K 116, 128
  betain 116
  folic acid 128–9, 139–40

Weed, Susun, *Menopausal Years. The Wise Woman's Way* 87
wild yam 86–7, 89, 98–9

xenoestrogens 95

yoga 177
  salute to the sun (suryanamaskar) 177, 222–3